Solution-Focused Nursing

Rethinking Practice

Edited by
Margaret McAllister

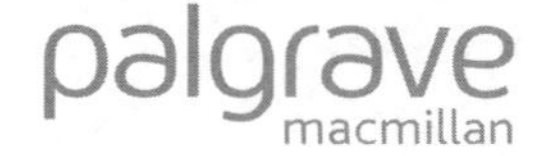

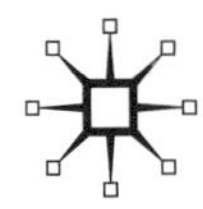

First published in 2007 by
PALGRAVE MACMILLAN
Houndmills, Basingstoke, Hampshire RG21 6XS and
175 Fifth Avenue, New York, N.Y. 10010
Companies and representatives throughout the world.

PALGRAVE MACMILLAN is the global academic imprint of the Palgrave Macmillan division of St. Martin's Press, LLC and of Palgrave Macmillan Ltd. Macmillan® is a registered trademark in the United States, United Kingdom and other countries. Palgrave is a registered trademark in the European Union and other countries.

ISBN-13: 978–1–4039–4627–0
ISBN-10: 1–4039–4627–2

This book is printed on paper suitable for recycling and made from fully managed and sustained forest sources.

A catalogue record for this book is available from the British Library.

10 9 8 7 6 5 4 3 2 1
16 15 14 13 12 11 10 09 08 07

Printed in China

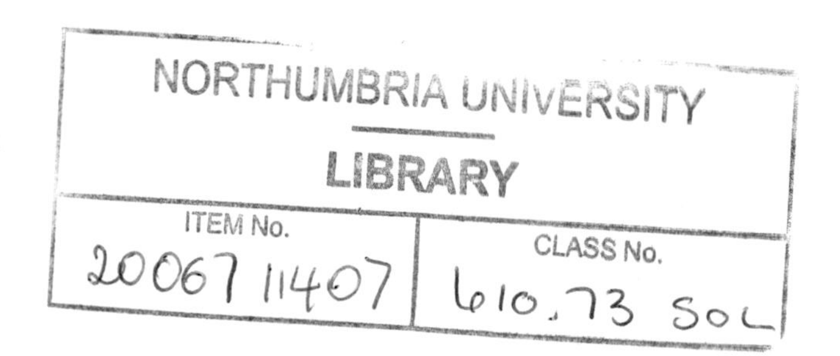

To my dear son Jimmy, who wants to be a writer too

Contents

List of Tables

Foreword

I want to raise two serious questions about nursing education and invite you the reader to reflect on them: Are schools of nursing continuing to prepare nurses for practice environments that no longer exist? And have conventional pedagogies in schools of nursing reached their use-by date, in terms of being able to respond to the industrialization of healthcare, the explosion of bioscience technologies and the move to community-based nursing care?

I argue that these challenges call for a change in the way nurses practice and consequently in the way they are taught. This text prompts a necessary rethinking of nursing practice. It opens the door for responding to changes in practice environments and simultaneously develops new pedagogies in schools of nursing. Solution-Focused Nursing offers a fundamental rethinking of nursing practice. It suggests a way to prepare nurses to meet the demands of contemporary practice environments.

As a teaching strategy, solution focused nursing attends to the dangers embedded in the current conventional pedagogies (outcomes and competency-based nursing education) and the focus in curricula on problem-solving and evidence-based nursing practice. It lays bare how a focus on problems and problem-solving can create an approach to nursing practice that is deficit-focused and bereft of an emphasis on strengths and possibilities. Problem-solving can hinder proactive, preemptive and preventive nursing actions that often embrace non-scientific, artistic and creative approaches. The strength of this book is its ability to bring solution focused counselling approaches into nursing in a way that preserves conventional approaches to nursing care, while overcoming limitations and creating visionary possibilities.

This book introduces students to solution focused nursing and a theory of nursing practice that avoids the dangers of the simple-to-complex and systems approaches, which result so often in an additive curricula. It utilizes Narrative Pedagogy to show students how solution focused nursing care includes evidence-based practice that is considered necessary but not sufficient. Compelling narratives are used that show alternatives to identifying client problems and matching these problems with best evidence-based nursing practice approaches. The solutions explicated by a variety of authors are thoughtful and thought-provoking. They proffer rich and thick narrative accounts to show students the complexities and necessity of exploring multi-perspectival thinking in the context of solution focus nursing care.

Perhaps the greatest strength of this book is the expertise of the authors in providing questions to guide the thinking of students and teachers as they together learn this new visionary rethinking of nursing practice. Solution-Focused Nursing does not require a dogmatic or prescriptive approach or the elimination of previous approaches to teaching nursing practice. Rather it is inclusive and embraces all possible ways of thinking, holding *all* approaches open and problematic. Instead of reproducing the conventional contexts for nursing care, for example acute care and community, this book shifts the focus to life transitions or those spaces where nurses actually conduct their practice. Throughout the book activities and questions engage the reader in a compelling exegesis of learning nursing practice.

This book offers a breath of fresh air to any teacher wanting to revise an introductory nursing course. The shift is from developing interpersonal and technical skill learning, to a focus on thinking in which voice is a central issue. The privileging of power is a central concern as the voices of clinicians and consumers resonate throughout the narratives. Faculties are experiencing challenges to better prepare students at all levels of nursing education. *Solution-Focused Nursing* provides a new theoretical approach that raises the bar by promoting an earlier I emphasis on learning critical and multi-perspectival thinking in the context of nursing practice. It advocates a different kind of nursing practice – one that is familiar and at-hand, yet radical and risky. The challenges to the dominant culture are significant while critical, feminist and post-structuralist theories guide a rethinking of nursing practice in transformative and visionary ways. If you never again want to teach a course on foundations for nursing, principles of nursing and nursing skills such as communication, this book is for you! Margaret McAllister and the authors of this book are to be commended for their stellar contribution to nursing literature and to rethinking practice through solution focused nursing.

Nancy Diekelmann PhD, RN, FAAN
University of Wisconsin – Madison
School of Nursing

Acknowledgements

Every attempt has been made to trace and acknowledge copyright, but in some cases this may not have been possible. The publisher apologises for any accidental infringements and would welcome any information to redress this situation.

Figure 1: A flash of Insight!. The image features Jimmy McAllister-Barnard and Aidan Hay. Taken on 12 June, 2005 and reproduced from the editor's own photographic collection.

Extract (on pp. 20–21) from *Atonement* by Ian McEwan 2001, published by Johnathon Cape, London. Used with permission of the Random House Group Limited

Figure 3: Analysing images on disability awareness Reproduced with permission from Paul Dicken, Director, Through the Roof. Registered charity no 1087788 PO Box 353, Epsom, UK

Song lyrics, p. 191, Hammer and a nail. By the Indigo Girls In *Nomads, Indians and Saints.* 2000, Audio cd. Sony.

Margaret McAllister would like to thank Darren Taggart, a student of the master of Mental Health Nursing, 2004, who provided the inspiration for the story in Chapter 7: 'Youth Work'. Names and other identifying features in the story have been changed.

She also wishes to acknowledge her gratitude towards her partner Jamie Hay, and friends Craig Shepperd, John Haberecht and Beth Matarasso who assisted her with Chapter 14: 'Helping Other People To Be Solution Focused' by sharing their teaching and caring expertise, and uplifting her with the deep and abiding humanism they show in their daily work and in their conversation with her.

Kenneth Walsh and Cheryle Moss, authors of Chapter 9: 'Solution Focused Mental Health Nursing', would like to acknowledge Professor Mary Fitzgerald of James Cook University, Cairns for her assistance in developing the group activity used within the chapter.

Notes on the Contributors

Trevor Adams, MSc, RMN, RGN, Cert Ed. CPN Cert. PhD, Lecturer in Mental Health, European Institute of Health and Medical Sciences, University of Surrey, Guildford, UK.

Margaret Barnes, RN, EM, BEd, MA, PhD, Senior Lecturer in Nursing, Faculty of Science, Health and Education, Sunshine Coast University, Queensland, Australia.

Bernie Carter, PhD, PGCE, BSc, RSCN, SRN, Professor of Children's Nursing, Department of Nursing, Faculty of Health, University of Central Lancashire, Preston, Lancashire, UK.

Michael Clinton, PhD, RMN, SRN, RN BA (Hons), FETeach Cert, RCNT, PGCert Ed, RNT, MSc, Faculties of Nursing and Medicine, University of Calgary, Canada.

Mary de Chesnay, RN, DSN, CS, FAAN Professor and N. Jean Bushman Endowed Chair, Seattle University College of Nursing, Seattle, WA, USA.

Anne Gardner, RN, PhD, Crit Care Cert, BA, MPH, PhD, Cabrini-Deakin Centre for Nursing Research, Deakin University and Cabrini Health, Victoria, Australia.

Glenn Gardner, RN, BAppSc(Advanced Nursing), MedSt, PhD, Professor of Clinical Nursing and Director, Centre for Clinical Nursing, Royal Brisbane & Women's Hospital and Queensland University of Technology, Australia.

Amanda Henderson, RN, RM, BSc, GradDipNurs(Ed), MScSoc, PhD, Nursing Director (Education), Princess Alexandra Hospital and Adjunct Associate Professor, Griffith University, Queensland, Australia.

Margaret McAllister, RN, RPN, Dip App Sci, BA, MEd, EdD, Associate Professor, School of Nursing and Midwifery, Research Centre for Clinical Practice Innovation, Griffith University, Queensland, Australia.

Paul Morrison, RN, PhD, RMN, BA (Hons), PGCE Grad Dip Counselling, AFBPS, CPsychol MAPS, Department of Nursing, School of Health Sciences, University of Canberra, ACT, Australia.

Cheryle Moss, RN, BappSc, MSc, GradDipEdAdmin, IAE, CCUCert, FRCNA, Graduate School of Nursing and Midwifery, Victoria University of Wellington, New Zealand.

Wendy Moyle, RN, Dip App Sci, BN (Ed.), MHSc, PhD, Professor, School of Nursing and Midwifery, Research Centre for Clinical Practice Innovation, Griffith University, Queensland, Australia.

Mike Musker, RMN, DPSN, BA (Hon), MSc, PGDE, Clinical Manager, Forensic mental health unit, South Australia, Australia.

Jennifer Rowe, RN, Dip Ed, BA, Grad Dip Ed, MPhil, PhD, Senior Lecturer, School of Nursing and Midwifery, Research Centre for Clinical Practice Innovation, Griffith University, Queensland, Australia.

Kenneth Walsh, RN, RPN, BNurs, PhD, Director, Nursing Research and Development Unit, Victoria University of Wellington and Waikato, New Zealand.

Introduction

This book discusses a new approach to nursing practice and a new nursing theory. Solution-Focussed Nursing is a practical philosophy, which emphasizes three things: the reasons to be cautious of dominant paradigms, a focus not only on problems but solutions too and strategies for working with and for clients, rather than on them.

In keeping with this subtle shift in emphasis towards solutions rather than problems within the problem-solving process, the book is structured, not around contexts of care (like hospital, community or home), which are usually dependent upon treatment or illness foci, but around life transitions. Life transitions are the spaces where nursing work is or should be most apparent. Nursing work in this space requires skilled helping that is not just technical, but also psychosocial and involves joining with a client, building their health and coping skills and extending those by engaging communities to assist so that adaptation, recovery, social connection and well-being are restored.

The view taken within this book is that critical education can help students to do nursing differently. Critical education is about students gaining knowledge and social relations that dignify one's own history, language and cultural traditions. It moves on from self-confirmation to the process by which students are able to interrogate and selectively appropriate those aspects of the dominant culture that will provide them with the basis for defining and transforming rather than serving, the wider social order (Giroux and McLaren, 1986, p. 318).

Our aims for you the reader, are to introduce you to a theory and practical approach that is being readily taken up within psychology, family therapy and business disciplines – the solutions focus – but which has so far not been widely discussed in nursing. We believe a solution orientation to problem-solving is valuable, and has potential to offer nursing and health care a way of working with clients that is more respectful, more optimistic and more enabling. We also want to impress upon you the value of developing a philosophy of nursing that is conscious of power and the ways culture can be reproduced and transformed.

For the literary world we hope that this book fills a gap. Most introductory nursing texts privilege the voice of the expert, focus on technical skills development and contain many recipes for practice. This book tries not to do that. Instead we include the voices of practicing nurses, real consumers (whose names have been changed) and stories that moved us to a new way of understanding and responding in the health sphere.

The book is divided into two sections. The first three chapters set the scene philosophically and practically. The idea is to convey practical theory drawn from critical, feminist and post-structural theories without overwhelming readers with complex information and by applying it to practice. The second section moves on to show how Solution-Focused Nursing can be applied in a variety of health transitions. In each chapter stories are told and analysed, readers are invited to engage in critical reflection, textual analysis and creative solution generating so that by the end of the book they may feel confident to apply the new knowledge and attributes in their own clinical environments. The book concludes with a chapter showing how readers might maintain their enthusiasm for being different (more solution-oriented, than problem centred) and go on to spread the word through teaching and research.

Solution-Focused Nursing shifts the emphasis on problem-solving to *solution searching* – a skill that requires creative, non-lateral thinking and partnership with clients to brainstorm ideas and try out novel approaches. We hope our readers are inspired to use the strategies we suggest, but also become creative producers of solutions of their own so that they may join us in advancing the specialty of nursing. Rather than focus on an individual and their problems, this book focuses on the individual in the context of a family, community and world and for whom the health-care aim is to develop healthy, peaceful, connected lives.

Margaret McAllister

Reference

Giroux, H. and McLaren, P. (1986). Teacher education and the politics of engagement: The case for democratic schooling. *Harvard Educational Review*, *56*(3), 213–238.

Please visit our companion website at www.palgrave.com/nursinghealth/mcallister to find resources to help lecturers integrate Solution-Focused Nursing into their teaching.

CHAPTER 1

An Introduction to Solution-Focused Nursing

Margaret McAllister

Overview

Imagine someone has lent you a pair of stilts and you've decided to wear them around the university campus for the whole day. You get to see things you don't normally see – books on the top shelves of the library, for example, and the tops of peoples' heads! From this perspective, the world looks altered somehow and your place within it is ever so slightly changed. Of course, everything within the world is actually still the same, but the way you relate to it is different. This is how it is with the solutions focused approach to problems.

Problems will still exist, and so too will the need for problem-solving, but the solution approach offers a different perspective to problems and problem-solving and illuminates new dimensions to issues so that you as a nurse, can approach clients' problems with fresh insight and creative ideas.

Basically the focus is on solutions not problems, the present and future, not the past and on what's going well or could be going well for clients rather than what's gone wrong.

Being Solution-Focused in Nursing

There are two key points to emphasize in explaining Solution-Focused Nursing. First, it concerns *solutions* and second it concerns *nursing*. Whilst it might seem obvious that health care workers ought to be working towards solutions to health care problems with clients, there is a very heavy emphasis in both policy and practice for clinicians to be problem-finders, rather than solution-searchers, and this argument will be illustrated and explained several times throughout the book. Furthermore, being good problem-finders does not necessarily mean that anything will change for clients and communities and this book and the model of SFN is all about emphasizing the importance of action. Without action, then models are reduced to empty theorizing.

So, Solution-Focused Nursing (SFN) aims to be a practical philosophy that uses multiple strategies to care for clients and moves beyond nurses being preoccupied with problems. It values both problem-solving and solution-searching so that problems can be identified and contained promptly, and solutions for restoring and maintaining health and well-being can be generated. Solution-Focused Nursing is interested in exploring and developing with clients their strengths and abilities rather than focussing solely on their weaknesses and disabilities.

Six Principles of SFN

1. The person, not the problem, is at the centre of inquiry.
2. Problems and strengths may be present at all times. Looking for and then developing inner strengths and resources will be affirming and assist in coping and adaptation. By working with what's going right with a client, one can be enhancing their hope, optimism and self-belief, thus maximizing their health capacity.
3. Resilience is as important as vulnerability.
4. The nurse's role moves beyond illness-care towards adaptation and recovery.
5. The goal is to create change at 3 levels: in the client, nursing and society. Thus it requires nurses to go beyond individual-focused care, to valuing the role of social and cultural care. It involves noticing practices that might be unhelpful or unjust and aiming to instead put in place empowering, enabling strategies. Understanding is not sufficient to enact change, one must be active, involved and committed.
6. The way of being with clients is proactive, rather than reactive. Care involves three phases of joining – or getting to know the person rather than the diagnosis; building, developing skills and resources the client can use to recover and adapt, and extending, opportunity for the client to practise these new skills and to connect with further social supports.

Why be Concerned with Developing Another Nursing Model?

There are now many different permutations of the solution orientation. It appears within business literature, in education and psychology but the model presented within this book has a distinct nursing flavour, hence the name Solution-Focused Nursing (SFN). In this age of interdisciplinarity, where borders between professions are merging, it is not always easy to distinguish between what is meant by Solution-Focused Nursing and what it means to be solution oriented in general. Indeed, some may argue that there is no need to delineate a separate identity for nursing work, but let me see if I can try to persuade you to believe my view that nursing does have a unique identity, though it shares borders with other groups, and perhaps why I think there is room and need for another nursing model.

I shall begin with a question. Can you, reader, answer this question honestly: Does nursing matter anymore? I don't mean does health care or medicine matter, for I'm sure we would agree that good quality health care is essential for any civilized society. I am asking a more discrete question: Does *nursing* really matter?

If you answered 'yes, I think it does', then I would argue that so too do nursing models. Nursing models help to articulate what nursing is, what nursing does, what nursing values and good nursing models illuminate the path ahead, helping nurses imagine and forge ahead to what nursing might become.

But if you answered 'Well, no I don't think nursing does matter anymore' ... Not in these post-modern times where we have moved beyond distinct professional boundaries and where what really matters is the care delivered, then we have a challenge ahead. For what my colleagues who contributed chapters in this book share is an optimism in the ongoing relevance of nursing and a belief in the distinctive qualities that define it. Each chapter offers various strategies that guide and extend nursing work, moving it beyond concern for the client's problem and towards assisting her/him to adapt, recover and find life meaningful in their health struggles.

Whilst authors in this book argue that there remains something unique and valuable about nursing, it does not mean that nursing should be permitted to flourish unchecked and uncriticized. For if nursing fails to be relevant to the communities it seeks to serve, then we do not deserve the trust placed in us. But this is exactly the point of developing a clear nursing model. In articulating our practice and our vision and then informing others about that, our accountability is raised and our possibility for contributing to social health and well-being is made that much more meaningful. The challenge, though, is to be convincing and clear so that new-comers and old-timers alike have their understanding, passion and commitment renewed.

How Does SFN Sit Alongside Existing Models?

Solution-Focused Nursing owes much to the nursing models that have come before and which sit alongside it. Nursing models have done much to progress nursing as a discipline and a culture because they attempt to articulate and define practice and practise ideals.

When we put into words the things we do and think, then the private realm is made public. This is a political act because it means individual practices can be transformed into collective action, an individual person's wisdom can be communicated so that others can understand and perhaps acquire it. The very culture itself, its language, rituals, history and values, has potential to strengthen and grow because that which was oral takes on concrete form and solid foundation. Whilst ever a culture is unstructured or unwritten it risks erosion and erasure. This is why good nursing models have practical value.

The process of putting into words that which we believe we do and think is itself influenced by prevailing discourses. *Humanism* is a world view that imbues Patricia Benner's model of Novice to Expert, *Interpersonal theory* shaped Hildegard Peplau's and Imogene King's models, a combination of *techno-rationalism* and *holism* influenced Virginia Henderson, Callista Roy and Dorothy Johnson and a movement away from science towards *new-age* influences the post-modern model proposed by Jean Watson. Thus not all models are the same. Points of difference arise precisely because of the world-views and assumptions about human nature and knowledge that underpin them. This is why it is important to discuss assumptions to SFN.

It is also possible that *differences* can exist alongside *shared* understandings. Simply because one model is different to another does not mean it stands against it in opposition. Contrary to what Glazer argues, when one is arguing for humanism, one doesn't necessarily argue against science (www.thepublicinterest.com/archives/2000summer/article1.html, 28 October 2005).

It is possible, as SFN is, to be both *for* humanism in the sense that it values each person's uniqueness and *for* science and what it can offer in the treatment of disease and the amelioration of suffering. Perhaps it differs from other models because it is less prescriptive or technical about how to assess and attend to the client's body. What it shares is a valuing of the contemplation of and theorising about nursing identity.

It is possible and important to continue theorising nursing. Seeking to understand identity/identities remains a worthwhile pursuit. Authors in this book do not subscribe to the pessimistic orthodoxy of some post-modernists who see an inevitable spiralling downward towards the proliferation of meaningless superficiality and thus the irrelevance of identity. Solution-Focused Nursing is a philosophy that aims to be as practical as it is idealistic. It believes that social justice is a realistic goal that can exist because of, not despite, the many differences that exist in this world. It understands that, as with life, not all health-care experiences will be perfect or problem-free, but as Peggy Chin (2002, p. 7) once said, 'the ideal, because it is imagined and envisioned, is possible'.

This is why it is argued in this book that nursing does have a distinct identity, even if and when it shares its borders with medicine and others. Nursing has discipline-specific knowledge with practice imperatives and a way of operating that are qualitatively different from all of the other health professions, but it is sometimes hard to articulate these differences. Even so, it remains important. Solution-Focused Nursing is one attempt to sketch out this unique profile.

Critics may desire and urge for more precision and detail to define Solution-Focused Nursing though this is resisted. As a practical philosophy, grounded in a diverse and shifting terrain it needs, at least for the moment, to be broadly based, sufficiently fluid to respond to local and emerging contexts of care, yet strengthened by clear values that illuminate the pathway ahead. These values are about being:

- For social justice. It supports the possibility for transformation in the client, in nursing and in society. It has a change agenda.
- For both/and thinking. This means that it values systematic and creative problem-solving, science and humanities, problem identification and solution generation.
- Alert to hidden binaries that set up an either/or mindset and thus excludes or minimizes the least advantaged position.
- Positioned with and for clients and to do that well, one needs to get to know who that individual client is, what their unique strengths and vulnerabilities are, what their goals and aspirations are. Expertise is therefore situated in both the nurse and the client. Each have something to share, and responsibilities to enact within the therapeutic relationship.

It is important to declare some assumptions about health and working with people that underpin this book. In doing this, an overarching world-view is made apparent, operating as a kind of pilot-light for how Solution-Focused Nursing, a philosophical model, might be lived out and developed.

Health and Well-being

To begin. The World Health Organisation (www.who.int) provides the following definition of health that is important to recall:

'Health is a state of complete physical, mental and social well-being and not merely the absence of disease or infirmity.' This means that health is more than that which might be located in one individual. Health is an ideal that, when it exists, encompasses all the functioning parts of a person – their mind, body, spirit, relationships and connections.

This may be a familiar concept to readers, but what may be novel is the point to follow. If we accept that health is all encompassing then why is it that we have so many clinicians who specialize in working with one body part and health services that service a body system rather than the whole person? As Donna Diers, a pioneer in the Nurse Practitioner movement in the United States said recently (2005), 'we should not be carving patients into small pieces'.

The fact that clients are distributed in health services in these ways is ideological. It shows us something about who has power to decide and what way of thinking is most highly valued. Clearly ideology and the dominant paradigm shapes how we think about these clients and how we interact with them. If wards are set up according to diagnoses, then problems become uppermost in the clinicians' minds. If we want to think in other ways, then it would be helpful to invent new ways of distributing clients. This requires a new mindset, structural change and new practices.

Herein, the philosophical assumption moves to action – nursing work involves working with the person and their communities and not just the presenting problem and not just by applying generic recipes and remedies.

Knowledge Needs to be Linked to Action

This leads to another important assumption, this time about knowledge. Knowing something and failing to take action is just empty theorizing. This is a world-view that resonates with feminists, critical social theorists, transformative teachers and environmental activists. So since we know, or at least assume, that health and well-being requires a holistic as well as individualized approach, nurses have a responsibility to be holistic, to be participatory, to enable people to articulate their own identities and concerns and to pursue a change agenda, through collective action.

Since holism joins the biological with the psychological, social and spiritual, there is no distinct border between the mind and the body, between the self and others. Each impacts upon the other.

We Live in a Changing World

At the social level this connection between previously separated concepts is part of what has been termed a post-modern age. This is where borders between countries, ideologies and professions are becoming more porous and diffuse. More people than ever have access to education, knowledge and communication. There is now greater awareness of differences existing amongst people so that one can no longer speak with certainty about what were once thought to be essential truths, about being a woman, for example or even a human being.

Indeed some beliefs are now considered tales that people simply told and retold, for example 'globalization', once thought to be a belief about free trade that would lead to a richer, freer more connected world for all, is now criticized as leading to some groups such as multi-national companies flourishing, whilst rural cultures are impoverished, there is more disconnection, marginalization and economic exclusion.

And in health care, the prevailing view once considered essential and thus told and retold through science, medicine and economics is that problem-centredness is the necessary approach. This issue will be examined and critiqued within following chapters.

For nurses, working in this changing world can be challenging. Nurses and nursing can sometimes feel lost or confused with the proliferation of ideas, concerns, differences and similarities. But it also offers enormous possibilities. With less firm boundaries between theoretical and practical divides, nurses are freer to cross borders and facilitate successful transitions for clients and their families, collaborate with new partners and broker support with new networks. It is a challenge to stay in touch with who you are and what you stand for when the world is in a state of flux, but it also means you can't easily stagnate. The future is uncertain but it is also exciting and new. Solution-Focused Nursing stems from these uncertainties and rather than attempting to rage against the present state of flux, aims to welcome change and value diversity.

Life Involves Health Transitions

Because people live in a constantly changing world, health maintenance can also be a continual challenge. Many changes that occur in a person's life may be related to life transitions – being born, adolescence, childbirth, menopause and old age. Sometimes, people need help to make successful passage across these transitions. Health care workers, especially nurses, can be crucial during this time.

Transitions Need Knowledge Workers

Transitions can be thought of like crossroads, points in a life journey where choices are made about which direction to take, which road to travel. Nurses are working at these transitions like border-workers, helping clients prepare well for their journey, explaining choices so that they can make informed decisions, working with them to build skills to enable them to make safe passage across sometimes shifting and difficult terrain. Notice that it is not about nurses taking away control, or doing things to people whether they like it or not. It is facilitative, participatory, respectful, acknowledging that sometimes people will make choices that the nurse may not make, that people do have their own priorities, pressures and values. How people act, live and see themselves is also shaped by the larger terrain or context in which they find themselves. As clinicians, nurses are an important part of that wider context for clients. While we are not responsible for the actions of others, we can be an influence. This is what is meant by being a transition worker.

Frequently the work of nurses is to interpret complex health information into language that the person understands, into sizes that are manageable and not overwhelming and into practices that can be taken up and used by the person in their everyday life. This is what is meant by nurses being knowledge workers.

Our actions, explored in this book – noticing strengths as well as vulnerabilities, reflecting on myths rather than working by habit, going beyond the biological to value the social and aiming to build not strip identities in people – can be the ripple effect for systemic and life-long change. It is a book that is fundamentally optimistic as this next assumption reveals.

Nurses Touch People

A simple sentence, just three words, but what depth lies in its potential.

There is a long and deep seated alliance between nursing and vulnerable people. Wherever you find individuals and groups that have fallen between the gaps of the health and welfare systems, who continue to experience substandard or even absent care, in those places nurses can soon be found. So, nursing has a valuable place in the human landscape. Where suffering occurs, succour and change is needed and so nurses can, perhaps should, be there.

Nurses occupy a distinctive place in the past, present and future and therefore continue to be valuable and ought to be valued in our health services and societies.

So there is something about Nursing's history that resonates with social-justice advocates and the discourses of critical social theory, difference theories and post-modernism. The vast majority of nurses are women and nursing is a gendered profession. Its voice is not sought, expressed, heeded or understood as clearly and as often as it could be. Nurses understand the position of marginalization and this offers potential for empathic engagement with individuals and groups who experience exclusion or alienation.

Nursing has long practised in ways that the context demands. When there are no doctors to care for rural populations, you will find nurses. Where shortages arise within health-care systems, nurses take on additional roles. They do this because they can. Nurses are shape-shifters, metamorphosing, filling gaps whenever and wherever the situation requires. Like other structures in society, nurses are diversifying, proliferating and transfiguring. This is our strength as well as our weak-point.

Having a primacy in practice has given nurses the precious reputation with clients as being trustworthy, accessible and reliable. Nursing isn't a discipline that risks reifying its knowledge and moving away from the human experience. It is dynamic and so has the potential to retain its relevance even if and when social policies and structures change.

Constant movement and blurred boundaries may keep the discipline dynamic and fresh. For some this means one no longer needs to think about one's nursing identity, what it means to be a nurse, for it is no longer relevant or important.

This diffusion can be read in another way though – that it is further splintering an already fragile, fractured group. There are now so many different role descriptors for practising nurses – the nurse-immuniser, the nurse-therapist and the nurse-endoscopist. At first glance, these titles may seem professionalizing and value-adding, but without a clear sense of identity (even if this is historical in nature only), these people risk being reduced to the specific function that they serve. Thus the question is posed: in whose interest is it to split nursing apart? Instead, one can take a passionate stance to argue that nursing's identity does have relevance, it is more than the current roles allocated to it. Since self-knowledge is crucial to self-development, theorizing about nursing's unique identity becomes an important tool for finding better ways to work towards social justice for the clients that it serves.

For some, nursing has an undervalued and undervaluing identity. There is evidence of residual and diffuse anger about this, about the seeming blind-spot that socializing agents such as media, politicians, schools and even families have towards nursing, which consequently perpetuates an out-dated, patronizing and limited scope for nurses.

Yet this anger grounds some nurses – keeping them fired up and determined to change peoples' minds, to shake up social ennui. Nurses are ever ready to fight against inequities or rules that are self-serving. The Nurse Practitioner movement across the world is a good example.

Collectively, though, nurses haven't been loud enough about disseminating achievements or in co-opting the media to help communicate our messages. There is more to do, more change to be made. This book outlines strategies that individually and collectively nurses can do to advance the change agenda.

But more than aiming to provide a range of solutions for nurses working in various health and life transitions, Solution-Focused Nursing aspires to offer meaning for nursing. Thus it is as philosophical as it is practical. Like other nursing models, SFN sees it important to reflect on and articulate nursing's identity. Reflecting on who 'we' are, and who we might want to include in our community, helps us decide what we seek and how well we are living the ideals of action and interaction that builds the kind of community that we actually want to achieve. So SFN aspires to be purposeful, practical and relevant.

Towards a Definition of Solution-Focused Nursing

Solution-Focused Nursing is a *philosophy* for nursing that guides the practice of nursing because it outlines ideals and values. It assumes that nursing work is, and can be, more than problem focused. It involves working with and for clients, so that health and well-being, meaning and life adaptation are promoted. This requires that students of nursing learn to move beyond a problem orientation.

Informed by post-modern and transformative world views, foregrounding difference and social justice, it aims to move disciplinary knowledge beyond understanding, towards committed action. In preparing for this, the student of Solution-Focused Nursing learns the skills of: critical thinking, consciousness raising and being with clients in positive solution-oriented ways.

It is these latter psycho-social skills that will be discussed in close detail within the pages of this book, primarily because of one final assumption: the current drive for scientific health care with its emphasis on empirical data and outcomes means that the artistic and expressive qualities of nursing are being undervalued and underutilized.

Why Practise Solution-Focused Nursing?

Practising Solution-Focused Nursing is an opportunity to correct the imbalance that exists within the health care system. There is a place for respectful, reflective and compassionate care that relies not on 'machines that go ping' or statistical data. Indeed these insights apply not just to person-centred care, but to management, education, leadership and research.

Insights and methodologies from social sciences notably metaphors, narrative therapy, solution-focused counselling, practice development, appreciative inquiry, action research and narrative inquiry are appropriated in this model to build strong, theoretically driven nursing interventions that can be used in any and all health care contexts. It is psychosocial nursing for every nurse.

From Where has Solution-Focused Nursing Emerged?

The solution focus is drawn from a number of different developments in thinking about change, clients, power and language. The positive psychology and family therapy movements are two places where the solution focus has been applied to therapy (Seligman, 1991; de Shazer and Berg, 1995). Linguistics, particularly post-structural theories that focus on the ways groups use language to set social agendas and assert or resist authority, often uses a solution focus to show how marginalized groups find new languages and solutions to resist being controlled (Foucault, 1980; Gilligan *et al.*, 1991).

While these disciplines are very different, they share the view that conventional and dominant ways of thinking about the world tend to focus on problems, and use reason and logic to understand them. In the therapy situation the tendency is to focus on disease and dis-comfort. In the social political situation, the tendency is to focus on dis-order and dis-empowerment. Both of these dominant practices tend to overlook what may be going well with clients and the world. A solution focus considers problems but focuses on ways of moving forward.

A Solution Focus Requires More than Technical Skills

Since the days of Florence Nightingale, nurses have known that their work involves much more than just reacting to problems. It involves prevention of problems, as well as actively developing strengths and abilities in clients during recovery and transition periods.

Learning to nurse also requires more than the mastery of skills of techniques, though these of course are important. It also involves the development of social and political awareness. In this book, we examine how nursing practice is a cultural practice – cultural practices are activities that shape how society functions, how it reproduces itself or how it changes.

To explain this important concept more clearly, it may be useful to think of race relations. The ways people from different races relate to each other is a cultural practice – it involves power, knowledge of difference, interpersonal skills and relationship between people. How well race relations take place within a community will influence how the culture of that community evolves.

Similarly, nursing involves power, knowledge of difference, interpersonal skills and a focus on relationship between people. How effectively this nursing/cultural practice operates will influence the ability of the health culture and the wider society to be responsive to all of its members. So learning to nurse, requires that students learn about nursing's place within society, learn to contribute to society in skilled and proficient ways and to contribute to visions for the future.

Major Assumptions about Social Change

Every theory is a social construct and thus it is important to reveal at the outset that there are some assumptions, which can not as yet be proven about Solution-Focused Nursing, but which nonetheless form the philosophy. Those assumptions are:

- There is no one right way of looking at things. Different views may be enriching and illuminating
- People are complex and unique and always have strengths as well as vulnerabilities
- Illness and wellness exist on a moving continuum. It is possible to have illness and suffering occurring in one aspect of a person and wellness and comfort in other areas
- The problem orientation is a dominant, mainstream and conventional approach to thinking. In practice this means that 'health care' is really 'illness care'
- Binary thinking is dominant in our society and ought to be questioned and reframed. problem/solution, illness/wellness, ability/disability, strength/weakness, us/them
- Helping strategies and health care professionals tend to be over-focused on searching for the cause of peoples' problems, when causes may not always be locatable
- Nursing care is crucial at every health transition and health transitions are not necessarily problem-states
- Nursing needs to move beyond the illness paradigm because it values proaction over reaction, coping over diagnosis and moving on over stabilization
- Small changes in the right direction can have a ripple effect, offering motivation and encouragement, hope and enthusiasm

So this list, which is likely to be incomplete because SFN is evolving and dynamic, are some beliefs that underpin the philosophy and which guide nurses acting in less problem-saturated ways, and in more capacity-building ways.

An important point to remember is that SFN is not pitted against other models. Individuals aspiring to SFN value that which has come before and realize that theories and practices are evolving. A problem orientation has many benefits, but has also been over-dominant in thinking and practice. SFN, too, may well have a use-by date because practical theory is not static. So, rather than think of SFN in opposition to problem-based nursing, it may be helpful to think of them as existing in concert. Sometimes it will be the trumpet's turn to sound and other times there is a place for violins. Let's turn our attention to the trumpet for a while so that we can appreciate its nuances and value.

The Problem Orientation

Thinking is an everyday mental activity that we use to process and understand information. While you and I might not spend much time thinking about thinking, there are many researchers, especially in psychology, who do. Those researchers have told us that problem-solving is one of the thinking skills that we use to help us to cope with novel situations and generate a suitable response (Myers, 1995). Some problems we solve by trial and error and others through logic and pattern making. Sometimes, we solve problems when an answer just comes to us in a flash of insight (see Figure 1.1). Problem-solving has also been called the scientific method, which involves some predictable stages and linear, deductive reasoning.

1. A problem is identified and described
2. Alternative solutions are considered
3. One solution is implemented and tested
4. The effects or results are evaluated.

In health care, the problem-solving method is crucial to the accurate identification of health problems, disorders and diseases. Health professionals learn how to be very good at being deductive, logical and rational so that they can carefully exclude problems that are not relevant and gradually isolate those problems that are. To solve problems effectively in health care one also needs to master the language of medicine. That is, health professionals need to understand physiology, anatomy, pathophysiology, diagnosis, pharmacology, palliative and restorative treatments.

In nursing, the scientific method has been appropriated and applied to health problems and is known as the Nursing Process. This is a logical and deductive approach, which helps to make sense of complex and multi-layered client issues. It involves standing back from the client and examining the problem(s), not the person. Through a process of systematic inquiry, health issues are

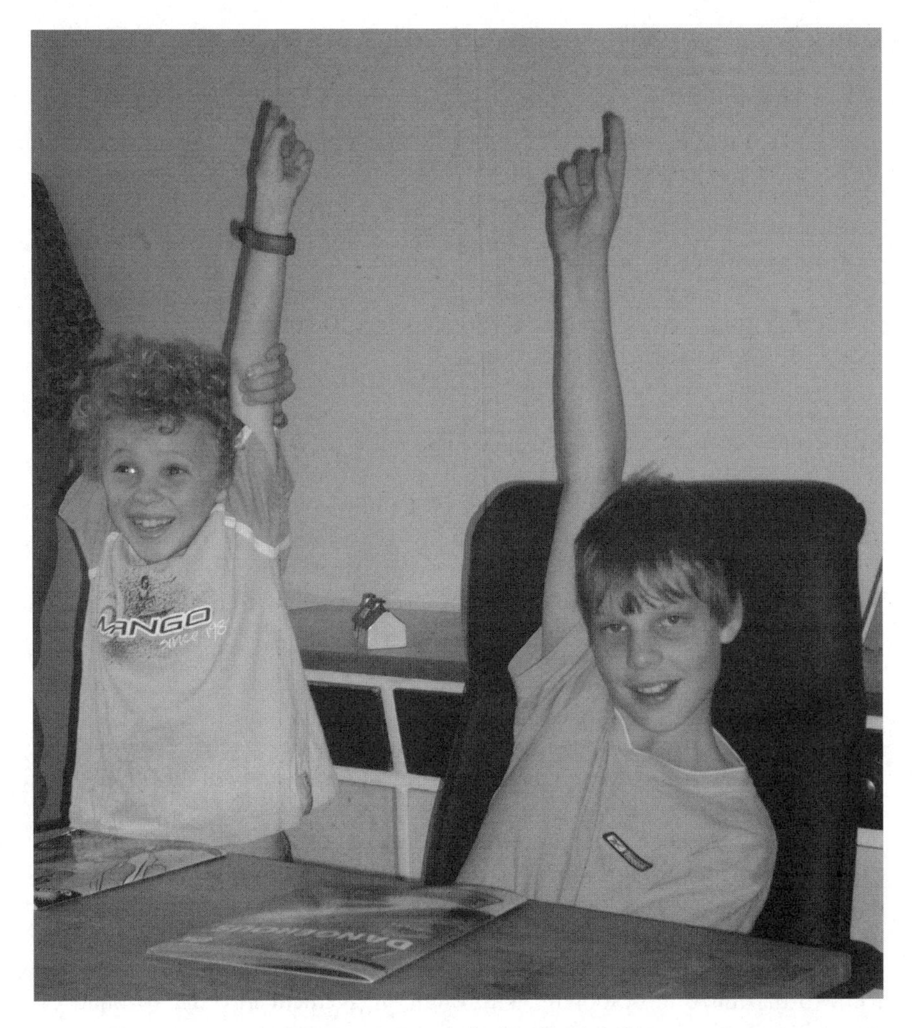

Figure 1.1 A flash of insight!

gradually eliminated until only the relevant problems for nursing work are left. Then, the nurse identifies possible solutions to this problem, selects one choice and implements it. Following a period of implementation, the nurse checks to see whether the strategy had the desired effect on the patient.

In this form of thinking, nurses tend to adopt a stance, which assumes:

- that the client (and their body) is in need, somehow deficient, perhaps resistant or lacking knowledge, ability or belief
- that the best way to think about problems is with logic and reason
- that the role of nurses and allied health is to assist medicine to make a diagnosis and provide treatment or remediation

- And in this form of thinking, nurses tend to perform a number of problem-oriented actions such as:
  - Asking the client/colleague what is wrong and why
  - Exploring historical causes and present difficulties in order to find a remedy
  - Searching for underlying issues to expose the 'real' problem
  - Elaborating on the experience of the client, rather than others in the social world
  - Label and categorize the client in problem-saturated ways
  - Focus on assessment of the client's problems and providing interventions
  - Privileging the health carer's voice and expertize
  - Use of specific professional jargon
  - Tending to be directive, strategic and sometimes mysterious

In the next chapter, you will explore in greater detail dominant views that shape how health care is practised, including the problem-orientation, pathology and diagnosis as well as new directions. Hopefully, you will come to appreciate the strengths and the limitations of these views and see the value in nurses becoming more active in employing strategies that move beyond an illness paradigm. And now let's look at how the violins sound within this concert.

The Solution-orientation

Unlike a problem orientation, a solution orientation doesn't simply identify and reveal difficulties. It also doesn't place the problem at the centre of the nurse-client interaction. A solution orientation acknowledges problem-solving as part of the nurse-client work, but foregrounds the presence of both problems and strengths. Like the problem-solving approach it is a form of clinical reasoning. But a solution-orientation involves logic and creativity, deductive and inductive thinking, imagination and reason, problem-solving and solution searching. A solution-orientation also works with what's going right with an individual or group, and seeks to maximize those potentials through engagement in order to build on strengths, achievements and capacity. In a solution orientation a nurse may:

- Ask what the client wants to change and how?
- Open spaces for future possibilities through a focus on exceptions and resources
- Invite a client to clarify main issues and priorities for health service
- Continuously channel a client and carer towards goals or desired actions
- Assume the client is competent, resilient and resourceful
- View a client as unique, and maintain a position of curiosity
- View nursing as interaction which opens new possibilities
- Focus on a process of collaborative inquiry
- Privilege the client's voice and expertise
- Build on a client's ideas and language
- Seek to be open, collaborative and respectful

Table 1.1 Problem-solving and solution orientations McAllister (2003)

Problem-solving method	*Solution Orientation*
• Health problems are central to the concerns of nurse and client	• Health problems are as important as healthy adaptation
• Aims to use the problem-solving method to understand and treat a client's problem	• Aims to understand problems and strengths, to promote resilience and health progresson
• Chooses problems over strengths	• Values both problems and strengths
• Logic and deductive thinking	• Deductive and inductive thinking
• Rationality	• Imagination and reason
• Remedial	• Creative
• Corrects deficits in lifestyle	• Reinforces present healthy lifestyle
• Diagnoses the problem	• Reframes problems to see it anew
• Motivates by giving plan of corrective action to follow	• Motivates by building on strengths, achievements and capacity
• Generates protocols and processes	• Generates personal plans and outcomes
• Health provider works on patient	• Health provider and client work together
• Provider prescribes conventional treatments	• Both people take reasonable risks to trial creative solutions

Searching for solutions requires imagination, creativity, abstract and lateral thinking. For some of us being creative is fun and exciting, but for others, it can be daunting. Mainstream society continues to value logic and reason, especially when it comes to serious work. But as you will see, there is a place for imaginative, creative play in nursing. Indeed it can be enriching, motivating and illuminating. Completing the exercises in each chapter may help you to uncover and exercise your imagination, building up your creative muscles so that you are more able to work with clients creatively and more likely to think about problems and solutions in novel ways. These are skills that will be useful to you throughout your life wherever you work.

From Shame to Pride: A Morality Tale for Nursing

About two years ago, I was lucky enough to have the chance to participate in a narrative research workshop where the class spent the whole day discussing the power of stories to convey insights not easily expressed in more 'scientific' techniques such as through graphs or reports. One of the facilitators for the day read out to us a story that not only encapsulated important elements of narrative, but somehow reminded me of the privileges and responsibilities of professional caring. I'll retell it here, and if you want to read it in its entirety the reference is at the end of this chapter.

A young girl named Minna and her family were poor mountain villagers who barely had enough money for food and shelter. Just as this story begins, her father, with whom Minna was very close, succumbed to chronic illness and died. The family struggled on and by winter, Minna was desperate to begin school, to join her friends and to learn new things. But in order to be able to attend, she had to have a warm coat.

Minna and her mother had no spare money and it seemed that all was lost. But then a friend from the village suggested that if everyone contributed one small rag from worn out clothes they no longer needed, then the quilting circle would make Minna the most beautifully warm coat that she could ever imagine.

The first day of school arrived and Minna proudly walked to school swinging and dancing about in her colourful coat. Even though the coat was made from rags, Minna knew that it was sewn from the love and generosity of all the people in her village. It made her recall something her father always used to say to her. 'All you need is people Minna. That's all you need'.

She went off to school happy and bright until some children in the playground began to scoff and tease her about the funny pile of rags she was wrapped up in. 'Rag Coat! Minna, you were better off with no coat than with that old, ragged thing' they laughed. But Minna didn't feel ashamed. Instead she showed them how the coat was not just rags, but made up of individual patches, sewn from peoples' favourite shirts, dresses and baby blankets, each with their own story to tell, each helping to keep her warm. And soon the children realized how lucky Minna was to have a coat made from the love of many people.

Reader Activity: Read Table 1.2 on the power of stories and reflect on the story above and these questions:

1. What morals or lessons for nursing can you find in this story?
2. How can 'the best' of nursing be compared with the community described in this story?
3. What does it mean for nurses to work with communities to support and extend care to clients?
4. How can you use narrative and imagery to help clients turn around a life problem into an opportunity?
5. What promise do you make now that will try to hear the voices of clients?

In some ways this story is not a typical health care tale. First, it is not about health or illness care. It is about a little girl struggling to feel safe, to belong to a group, and to accept support. It is about courage, difference and acceptance. It's about creative problem-solving and turning crises into turning points.

Table 1.2 The power of stories

1. Stories are able to evoke and transmit feelings, thereby allowing other people to relate to them
2. One can become immersed in a good story (events become personal to us, it is harder to be detached, and thus more likely to be more people to care, to remember and to act)
3. Language is the great transmitter of culture, we can share cultural lessons through language, and thus strengthen, advance and share understanding of that culture
4. In stories, context is emphasized and this is important, because nursing practice can't be understood without context. Our practices change depending on context, and no single rule applies
5. When we speak in public forums, this is potentially a political act because it shares information, connects people and can change peoples' views. Stories, publicly told, are ways for nurses to be political.

So, the little girl can be seen as a metaphor for all clients. Perhaps the strengths, challenges and resources differ for each person, but there are some human needs that we all share. And the village folk might be the health care team, resourceful, creative problem solvers, engaged in collaborative support.

Another way that this is not a typical story of health care is that it is a story about empowerment, about the community coming together to work towards a solution. Unfortunately, the more common story is that which features people (also referred to as patients, service users or clients) experiencing ongoing suffering, being patronized, marginalized or receiving inadequate care. There are also many stories of nurses being hurried, overworked, underpaid, ignored and overlooked. These common stories are often told, but in their frequent telling, less common stories remain untold. When we recall more positive experiences, and bring them to the forefront we may be able to see signs of hope, other pathways, more choices and another way of being and doing nursing.

That is why this book will relay more uncommon stories, stories which contain within them some lessons that point towards ways of being solution-oriented. Reading between the lines, you may begin to understand why tales of domination, exclusion and unhappiness have tended to recur for nurses and clients, as well as illuminate alternative approaches. New solutions can become apparent when we look at issues armed with new frameworks or creative ideas. So instead of surrendering to the inevitable view that health environments will always function as 'illness care' places we will take a more optimistic view.

The next chapter exposes some of the leading, dominant health discourses, which can reduce our optimism about change in nursing and health care. These discourses are commonly apparent in language, social practices and public images. They are heard and seen in advertising, television, movies and books and continue to link nursing with disorder and disease. These dominant discourses are not particularly relevant to most nurses or patients and they have a marginalizing effect, making clients feel insecure, stupid, angry or afraid. They also tempt nurses to use power over clients, and to see themselves as 'us' and clients as 'them'. But there are different ways. The challenge for we the writers and you the reader, is to reveal them.

Suggestions for Further Readings

Furman, B., and Ahola, T. (1992). *Solution talk.* Norton: New York.

Gingerich, W., & Eisengart, S. (2000). Solution-focused brief therapy: A review of the outcome research. *Family Process, 39*: 477–498.

McAllister, M. (2003). Doing practice differently: Solution-Focused Nursing. *Journal of Advanced Nursing. 41*(6), 528–535.

Mills, L. (1991). *The rag coat.* Boston: Little Brown and Co.

O'Hanlon, B. (1999). *Do one thing different.* New York: William Morrow.

Wilkin, P. (2001). The other side. *Mental Health Nursing, 21*(5), 28. Retrieved 11 February 2002 from the world wide web: http://proquest.umi.com/pqdlink

Teacher notes to accompany this chapter can be found at www.palgrave.com/nursinghealth/mcallister

CHAPTER 2

Cultural Roots and New Developments in Nursing

Michael Clinton

Overview

This chapter will introduce and explain concepts that will help you to understand the theoretical context in which Solution-Focused Nursing is emerging, including:

- How theory is used in Solution-Focused Nursing discourse
- Clarification of concepts in post-modernism
- Discourse analysis
- Concepts of power, ideology and hegemony
- Freedom, power and resistance
- Transformational thinking as a means to emancipation
- Emancipation and the empowerment of patients, clients and families
- Reflexivity in post-modern thought and Solution-Focused Nursing

Over the years nurses and nursing have been extended and constrained by dominant discourses. We have already briefly mentioned Florence Nightingale, and readers will no doubt appreciate the enormous influence both she and the hygiene movement of which she was a part, had for nursing in the western world. Another huge influence over the ways nursing was to develop came in the war years, particularly the Second World War. Take a look at this excerpt from Ian McEwan's (2001) novel *Atonement.*

> Briony's state of mind largely depended on how she stood that hour in the ward sister's opinion. She felt a coolness in her stomach whenever Sister Drummond's gaze fell on her. It was impossible to know whether you had done well. Briony dreaded her bad opinion. Praise was unheard of. The best one could hope for was indifference.
>
> ... Briony had thought she was joining the war effort. In fact, she had narrowed her life to a relationship with a woman fifteen years older who assumed a power over her greater than that of a mother over an infant.

This narrowing, which was above all a stripping away of identity, began weeks before she had even heard of Sister Drummond. On her first day of the two months' preliminary training, Briony's humiliation in front of the class had been instructive. This was how it was going to be. She had gone up to the sister to point out courteously that a mistake had been made with her name badge. She was B. Tallis, not, as it said on the little rectangular brooch, N. Tallis.

The reply was calm. 'You are, and will remain, as you have been designated. Your Christian name is of no interest to me. Now kindly sit down, Nurse Tallis.'

... Briony already sensed that the parallel life, which she could imagine so easily from her visits to Cambridge as a child to see Leon and Cecilia, would soon begin to diverge from her own. This was her student life now, these four years, this enveloping regime, and she had no will, no freedom to leave. She was abandoning herself to a life of strictures, rules, obedience, housework, and a constant fear of disapproval. She was one of a batch of probationers – there was a new intake every few months – and she had no identity beyond her badge. There were no tutorials here, no one losing sleep over the precise course of her intellectual development. She emptied and sluiced the bedpans, swept and polished floors, made cocoa and Bovril, fetched and carried – and was delivered from introspection (pp. 274–6).

From Atonement by Ian McEwan, published by Jonathan Cape. Reprinted by permission of the Random House Group Ltd.

Adherence to military order, rules, obedience, sacrifice and duty are clearly fore-grounded in this text and indeed are characteristics that continue to be revealed in many nursing practices today. Certainly during times of war, such attributes are necessary for efficiency and control, but they come at a cost.

Reader Activity: Make a list of the attributes identified in McEwan's story that you think were positive for the health care system and negative for the nurse's identity

Describe any evidence of concepts listed in the overview

Imagine that you were a student of nursing during this time. What interpersonal skills might have assisted you in surviving, or perhaps influencing, the process of care?

What theories (biological, social, political or psychological) might have been informative for you?

By analysing McEwan's story for what it says positively and negatively about nursing, you have engaged in a theoretical process called Discourse Analysis This use of theory helps to delve deeply into a practice, and see things that you might not otherwise see about how cultures such as nursing, are shaped. This chapter will now go on to examine the emergence of Discourse Analysis and other theoretical ideas more closely.

If you were to look up the definition of the word 'theory' in any English dictionary you are likely to find a definition that includes the following or similar phrases:

(a) A supposition or a system of ideas intended to explain something, especially one based on general principles independent of the thing to be explained
(b) An idea accounting for or justifying something
(c) A set of principles on which an activity is based (*The Concise Oxford Dictionary*, 1999).

Theories are not just relevant to nursing work, they are crucial, because they help us to be conscious about our practice rather than unconscious. When we are unconscious, like poor Briony, the character in McEwan's novel, who has been 'delivered from introspection', we carry out procedures in boring repetition, in soul-destroying half-heartedness, in ways that can be cold, uncaring and even cruel. In short, theories help us to use what is relevant and discard what no longer helps us to be caring.

Reader Activity: Browse through Part Two of this book. Write down the numbers of the chapters that interest you most in the first column of Table 2.1. Put the names of the authors in the next column. In the third column, put in the letter that corresponds to the phrase that best indicates how the authors use theory to discuss Solution-Focused Nursing. That is, for each chapter indicate on the basis of your first impression whether the authors: (a) present a system of ideas independent of Solution-Focused Nursing, (b) account for and/or justify Solution-Focused Nursing, or (c) provide principles for putting Solution-Focused Nursing into practice. (You can put more than one letter against the names of the authors if you like.)

Now look back at Chapter 1. You will see that Margaret McAllister gives an overview of Solution-Focused Nursing that fits well, but not exclusively, with the third phrase in our definition of theory, phrase c. What about the other contributors to this book? How, for example, do the authors of Chapters 4, 6 and 11, use theory in their chapters? How am I using theory in this chapter? These are important questions to ask. Why? Because the 'new developments' referred to the title to this chapter concern how theory is used. A harder question to answer is whether any of the chapters, including this one, amount to a system of ideas that is independent of Solution-Focused Nursing.

Reader Activity: Reflect on the thoughts that led to your entries in Table 2.1. Take a few minutes for this. Then write down notes in answer to this question: How is the phrase (a) above different from phrases (b) and (c)? Clue: Re-read the final sentence in the previous section.

Table 2.1 Uses of theory exercise

Chapter	*Author(s)*	*Phrase (a, b, c)*

Theorizing Solution-Focused Nursing

You are thinking along the right lines (or at least in the same way I am) if you noted use of the concept of 'independence' in phrase a) because there is nothing in phrases b) or c) that suggests a theory can be independent of its applications. This brings us to two ways of thinking about theory and Solution-Focused Nursing: the first is associated with ideas often called modernism; the second with post-modernism.

These terms might be new to you, so let us try to get clear about them.

Modernism

In philosophy, modernism is taken to be the train of thought that began with Descartes (1596–1650) and seeks to lift human reason to a level immune from doubt. In more recent times, modernism is understood as the intellectual movement, sometimes called The Enlightenment that sees mathematics, logic and empirical science as the means of freeing human thinking from ignorance and superstition. As a result, a characteristic feature of modernism is its close association with positivism.

Positivism

Positivism is now understood as meaning just about the same thing as empiricism – the idea that we can only find out what can be known by using our five senses, augmented as necessary by instruments of various kinds, such as electroencephalographs and Magnetic Resonance Imaging. But originally, the French sociologist, historian and philosopher Comte (1798–1851) coined the term positivism to describe the stage in history when human thought itself became a subject for science. However, a dominant tendency in Comte's thought was to think of the sciences in hierarchical order, with astronomy and physics at the top, followed in order of precedence by the biological, human and social sciences. Note that the reason why Comte gave precedence to some sciences over others was because those he rated more highly were those that involve theories that exemplify our phrase a) definition. That is, the most prestigious sciences are those that involve complex mathematical reasoning that is independent of their subject matter.

Post-modernism

Post-modernism is a general term used to refer to a broad range of social movements and cultural trends, from architecture to literature and philosophy, which share a preference for a variety of ways of thinking rather than acceptance of such claims as:

1. Science is independent of its subject matter
2. There are fundamental and inalienable truths for science to discover, and that
3. Positivist thinking can be applied to human thought

The two features of post-modern thinking that are most relevant to this chapter are its linguistic turn and its concern for self-reflexivity. The term 'linguistic turn' refers to post-modern thinkers' preoccupation with language and how it is used, which is why we started with definitional phrases of 'theory'. Self-reflexivity is the relationship human thinking has to itself, including the kinds of practices encouraged in Chapter 3.

Discourse Analysis

Post-modern thinkers such as Michel Foucault (1926–1984) prefer the term discourse to language. This is because they make an effort to understand how language is used, including what is passed over or taken for granted in the way we speak to one another and write down our thoughts for others to read. Of particular concern to Foucault was the relationship between:

- Language use and the social and spatial location of users
- Discourse and socialization
- Language use and ways of living
- Language use, power and ideology
- Freedom, power and resistance

These concepts will be clarified, but for the moment note that in post-modern thought the process of examining relationships of this kind is called discourse analysis.

Let us try some discourse analysis.

Read the following short section taken from Florence Nightingale's (1820–1910) *Notes on Nursing*, first published in 1859.

> No mockery in the world is so hollow as the advice showered upon the sick. It is of no use for the sick to say anything, for what the adviser wants is not to know the truth about the state of the patient, but to turn whatever the sick may say to the support of his own argument, set forth, it must be repeated, without any inquiry whatever into the patient's real condition. 'But it would be impertinent or indecent in me to make such an inquiry,' says the adviser. True; and how much more impertinent is it to give your advice when you can know nothing about the truth, and admit you could not inquire into it. (www. digital.library.upenn.edu)

Note the connection between Florence Nightingale's main point and Solution-Focused Nursing. Nightingale is advising that everyone, including nurses, should avoid giving advice to 'the sick' because we cannot possibly know their 'real condition'. However, note that Nightingale stops short of telling us that we should help 'the sick' to draw on their strengths to solve problems. In other words, both Nightingale and Solution-Focused Nursing advocate not imposing our views on 'the sick' (read patients, clients and families) but Nightingale stops short of advising nurses to find out what patients' strengths are in order to help them solve problems. Why? Because for Perhaps you can investigate why this might be so in the following Reader activity.

Reader Activity: Read through Nightingale's Notes on Nursing on-line and write down ten possible reasons based on the values of Victorian Britain and the place of (high born) women in Victorian society. The process you use to identify these reasons is a form of discourse analysis.

Reasons why Nightingale thought it impertinent for nurses (or anyone else) to ask 'the sick' about their 'real condition':

1.
2.
3.
4.
5.

Relate as many of your points as you can to the following:

1. The social location of Nightingale as a high born women writing in the London of the mid 1850s.
2. Nightingale's socialization as a woman familiar with the manners and demeanour of her class.

3. The life style wealthy families would have enjoyed in Nightingale's day (Clue refer what Nightingale says about servants, and focus on the implications for nursing)

We think very differently about working with patients, clients and families now, which is why Solution-Focused Nursing is receiving increasing attention.

Historical Transitions

A good way to understand why ideas about nursing change is to read the thoughts of nurse theorists. Consider the following summary of a paragraph written by Jean Watson, Professor of Nursing at the Center for Human Caring, University of Colorado:

The post-modern turn in the history of nursing is hallmarked by the fact that the knowledge that has been systematically excluded from the human consciousness now has to be restored and reconnected in order to reconnect with the human condition (Smith, 1982). Some of that knowledge is knowledge of what it means to be human that goes beyond the physicalist, material orientation and fixation of the modern era. Part of that knowledge is an awakening of nursing's moral consciousness and compassion that moves in concentric circles and chains (Noddings, 1984), from self care, to caring for others, to environment, to nature, to caring for and being part of an evolving universe that people are cocreating (1999, p. 475).

Watson's first sentence is concerned with the kind of knowledge that Nightingale explicitly excludes when she states that it would be impertinent to ask about the 'patient's real condition'. Watson also makes a broader point in that she argues for connecting our understanding of the 'patient's real condition' with a deeper appreciation of 'human consciousness' and the 'human condition'. Her point is quite general because she is looking past nursing to an ethical and compassionate way of thinking that is beyond modernity. Hence, Watson disparages the limitations of positivist science to advocate for a holistic way of thinking that is more capable of encompassing the human dilemmas of today. This is made clear in the final sentence, when Watson stresses a point directly relevant to Solution-Focused Nursing. Note that Watson situates 'caring' in a realm of meaning that is cocreated (created in unison with) those we care for as nurses. Moreover, Watson's connects the cocreation that occurs between the individual 'patient' and nurse with the concurrent cocreation of a wider universe of meaning, in which it becomes possible to understand what it means to be a person.

Note also that Watson:

1. Puts knowledge of the human condition in general as the focal point of human caring.
2. Implies that nurses should connect their understanding of the particular patient, client or family and of themselves with this broader conception

3. Regards physicalism (the notion that positivism is capable of identifying a material basis for all scientific phenomena) as an incomplete basis for understanding the problems of today.
4. Seeks to awaken the moral conscience and compassion of nursing that is excluded from the kind of understanding that is associated with science and technology.
5. Advocates for radical transitions in nursing's concerns and practice.
6. Requires that nurses see themselves and those they work with as co-operating in the construction of universal meanings that reflect the human condition.

In other words, Watson wants to:

- Replace the precise knowledge of science with toleration of ambiguity
- Find a place for poetry, aesthetics and imagination in nursing practice
- Foster thinking that emancipates nurses and empowers those they work with
- Focus the attention of nurses on the lived reality of nursing and nursing practice
- Find a way of understanding nursing that has human authenticity rather than scientific validity
- Focus on processes, transitions and transformations, rather than on social structures such as hierarchies and organizations
- Elevate the relevance of meaning above that of factual claims
- Elevate spiritual ways of thinking and being above contemporary materialism and selfish values (Watson, 1999, p. 476).

Reader Activity: Complete Table 2.2 by identifying resonances of Watson's thinking in the accounts of Solution-Focused Nursing in Part Two of this book.

When you have finished this activity answer the following questions:

1. What do post-modern thinking about nursing and justifications of Solution-Focused Nursing have in common?
2. Is there anything about Solution-Focused Nursing that is inconsistent with Watson's post-modern thinking?

Power, Ideology and Hegemony

Three concepts help us to better understand the resonances of Watson's thinking in Solution-Focused Nursing.

Table 2.2 Resonances of Watson's thinking in Solution-Focused Nursing

Watson's transitions to:	*Resonance in SFN*	*Chapter number*
Tolerance of ambiguity		
Use of poetry, aesthetics and imagination in nursing practice		
Emancipation of nurses		
Empowerment of patients, clients, families		
Lived realities of nursing and nursing practice		
Focus on human authenticity		
Focus on processes, transitions and transformations		
Privilege meaning over empirical facts		
Elevate spirituality above contemporary materialism and selfish values		

Power

Watson's advocacy of transitions in nursing calls into question the power arrangements that work in favour of the status quo. However, it is important to understand the distinctly post-modern interpretation of power that Watson implies. According to Foucault, power is not something that is possessed by individuals and deliberately exercised over others. Rather power is a complex and widely diffused phenomenon that has indeterminate effects. In other words, the outcome of power relations is always a contingent matter because people are not and cannot be aware of all of its operations and implications. This lack of awareness partly explains why power relations continue, and why change in nursing involves consciousness raising as well as the transformation of practice.

It is important to note that for Foucault, knowledge and power are closely related because power relationships are implicit in knowledge, and uses of knowledge involve the exercise of power. However, power relationships never work in one direction only because those who may be regarded as subject to it are free to resist, without always being aware that this is the case. This is why, when doing a discourse analysis on cultural practice, it is important to notice sites of resistance, for these are spaces where power and its reproduction may be being resisted and changed.

Watson's writing provides an important example in that she wants to overcome the limitations on nursing practice that are imposed by a purely scientific (read empirical) view of nursing. Empirical knowledge will always be highly influential in nursing, but Watson shows that empiricism is incapable of helping us to understand what she calls 'the human condition'. In other words, Watson is subjected to the same dominance of scientific thinking as the rest of us, but she is able to raise our awareness to a level at which we can see why it is important to put scientific knowledge into a broader and more critical perspective.

Ideology

There is a close relationship between the concept of power and that of ideology. Ideology refers to a collection of beliefs and practices that serve other than epistemic purposes for those that have them. For example, scientific knowledge not only reflects the discoveries of science, but incorporates beliefs about:

- What sort of science is important
- How science should be and is conducted (not always the same thing)
- The supposed value-neutrality of science
- The status of scientists as experts
- The precedence scientific language over other kinds of discourse

The epistemic interests of scientists are those that are concerned with what can be known and are based (for the most part) on reasoning to the best explanation of empirical data. However, critiques of scientism, such as those implicit in Watson's views are no less ideological as in post-modernism there can be no ideological free knowledge because all knowledge is associated with the interests of those who profess it. For example, Watson's view that science can provide only a partial view of nursing that stands in need of transcendence by a more humanistic account is a style of criticism that is based on its own values and beliefs, particularly those associated with feminist theory. This is not to criticize Watson, but to point out that every time we claim to know something on the basis of a theoretical standpoint, we rely on antecedents that can themselves be subjected to ideological critique. The 'hallmark' of such critiques, to use one of Watson's words, is that they seek to invert one reality in favour of another. The reality that Watson inverts is that of scientism in favour of her brand of humanism, which is not a bad thing, merely an expression of a different and, perhaps, better (in some sense) ideology. The realities of modernism and its inversions in post-modern thinking are the cultural roots in the title of this chapter.

Hegemony

The concept of hegemony refers to ideas that have become so dominant that they are taken to be natural and they usually defy, or at least escape, criticism.

The key idea is that some ways of thinking reflect the ideas of dominant groups that exert leadership over morality and intellectual movements. Originally developed as part of Marxist (in the tradition of the thinking of Karl Marx 1818–1883) critiques of capitalism, the concept of hegemony is now more broadly applied to refer to the ways in which the ideas of dominant groups are perpetuated and reproduced through processes of socialization, especially in schools, in the workforce, and in preparation for the professions. In nursing, it has become commonplace to criticise the hegemony of positivist science and the paternalism that is associated with some kinds of medical practice. Therefore, overcoming the hegemony of science and the medical model in health care has become a preoccupation of nursing theorists.

Two Discourses on Socialization

The concepts of power, ideology and hegemony provide us with two different views on the socialization of nurses. In the first view, which I shall call the traditional view, nurses are in danger of being narrowed by their professional preparation by being socialized into power relations, ideologies and hegemonic assumptions that are inimical to their status as health professionals. On the alternative view, which I shall call the emancipated view, nurses are capable of knowledge that overcomes all of the most serious impediments to their emancipation – positivism, scientism, materialism, paternalism and secularism are all inverted in the service of the cocreation of more inclusive ideological order. However, it is a basic tenet of the emancipated view that the emancipation of nurses is not only important for its own sake, but also for the empowerment it can bring to patients, clients and families. In other words, the emancipated view is concerned to socialize nurses into recognizing the importance of supporting the freedom of those they work with by empowering them to make their own decisions, even when they are contrary to established power relations and hegemonic practices. Hence, the importance of Solution-Focused Nursing as a new direction for nursing practices.

Conclusion

This chapter has introduced theoretical notions important to understanding and critiquing Solution-Focused Nursing. Developing out of the post-modern turn in philosophy and social science, SFN is underpinned by assumptions about power and how it can be reproduced or resisted, how it can be used to dominate or emancipate, how the culture of nursing is reproduced but how it can be transformed by noticing and perhaps supporting various sites of resistance.

Contemporary cultural theories in post structuralism and feminism are developing concepts such as care, culture, and practice within contemporary nursing so that currently these concepts are not just defined but are being theorized and developed as part of the discipline of knowledge in nursing. The renewed focus on multiple knowledges, local contexts and interconnections is seeing a resurgence of theory linked with practice. It reminds students that power can be shared, there are alternatives to mainstream practices, and scientific knowledge can not on its own, produce comprehensive health care. Nursing needs to discuss and develop ways of working with and for clients, using creativity and reason.

The chapter has also emphasized the importance of being conscious of subtle practices and beliefs that are shaping or attempting to shape nurses and nursing.

Suggestions for Further Reading

Clinton, M. and Nelson, S. (1999). Recovery and mental illness. In Michael Clinton and Sioban Nelson (eds), *Advanced practice in mental health nursing*. Oxford: Blackwell Science.

Cutting, G. (1994). *The Cambridge companion to Foucault*. Cambridge: Cambridge University Press.

Rodgers, B. (2005). *Developing nursing knowledge: Philosophical traditions and influences*. Philadelphia: Lippincott Williams & Wilkins.

Watson, J. (1979). *Nursing: The philosophy and science of caring*. Boston: Little Brown.

Teacher notes to accompany this chapter can be found at www.palgrave.com/nursinghealth/mcallister

References

Gee, J. (1987). What is literacy? *Teaching and Learning, 2*, 3–11.

Gee, J. (1999). *Social linguistics and literacy*. New York: Taylor & Francis.

Nightingale, F. *Notes on nursing*. Accessed on the internet at: http://digital.library.upenn.edu/women/nightingale/nursing/nursing.html#XIII, sighted 21 February, 2005.

Noddings, N. (1984). *Caring: A feminine approach to ethics and moral development*. Berkeley: University of California Press.

Smith, H. (1982). *Beyond the post-modern mind*. Wheaton, Illinois: Theosophical Publishing House.

Watson, J. (1996). Watson's theory of transpersonal caring. In J.Fitzpatrick and A.Whall (eds) *Blueprint for use of nursing models: Education, research, practice and administration*. (pp. 141–184). New York: National League for Nursing.

Watson, J. (1999). Postmodernism and Knowledge Development in Nursing. in E. Carol Polifroni and Marylouise Welch (eds), *Perspectives on Philosophy of Science in Nursing: An Historical and Contemporary Anthology*.(pp. 471–77). Philadelphia: Lippincott.

CHAPTER 3

The Spirit of SFN: Making Change at Three Levels

Margaret McAllister

Overview

This chapter will explain and apply important theoretical aspects of Solution-Focused Nursing:

- Nurses are transition workers: proactively joining, building and extending care for clients
- It highlights ways of thinking that constrain the culture of nursing, and help to transform it
- A focus on interpersonal, social and cultural levels
- At the interpersonal level skills to be developed are in joining with the client, using questions strategically in order to notice strengths and build hope
  - Clarifying values and critical reflection: Two ways to bring to the surface those concepts and ideologies that have been taken-for-granted and no longer noticed, but which can lead to change and empowerment
  - Strengths focused assessment
- At the social level, skills to be developed are in raising consciousness about nursing, building solidarity and changing oppressive rules and conditions which constrain nursing
- At the cultural level, skills to be developed are in raising public awareness of the contributions and developments in modern nursing and in motivating the profession to become active in every-day empowerment politics

Introduction

This chapter explores the spirit of Solution-Focused Nursing. In other books on nursing you might read about philosophy, principles or practices. This chapter discusses all of those things but in ways that are grounded in the every-day. In this way, you will hopefully see that there is no one 'how to' in nursing, but many ways to approach issues, and come to share my view that there's nothing as practical as good theory.

You will be introduced to some insights and cognitive skills, which may be new to you. And you might find some of it surprising. You may think 'but what's this got to do with nursing?' – Especially if you are still thinking that to be a nurse, all you need is physical strength and common sense. But try to hang in there, because by the close of the chapter you will have developed at least five essential thinking skills that will help you understand and practise nursing with critical awareness. And this critical awareness is what we need to change practice, to advance health care. If you learn these concepts and apply them daily, you will become important for positive change tomorrow.

Surfacing, Clarifying, Crystallizing Values

If you were to ask members of the public what they expected a good nurse to be like, what do you think they'd say? Imagine what your parent, brother or sister might say and write down their answer here. To make a start, I've recorded what my young son suggested.

- They'd be nice to people, they'd be helpful and efficient.
- ...
- ...

Take a look at all the descriptors inserted now into the box above and see if you can identify a common theme. Is it about helpfulness, kindness, efficiency? These are all true enough, but they don't really explain how nursing might differ from all other human service workers, like child care workers, aged care workers or even supermarket check-out operators.

Reader Activity: Try this one minute activity. Without thinking too much, write down all of the values that you believe a good nurse could hold.
Compare your answers with the values apparent in the previous activity. What are the similarities and differences?

Spending time clarifying the personal values you hold and merging them with the professional values espoused by the discipline of nursing is an important challenge for you as you make the transition from lay person to professional.

Not all of us regularly think about the values of the profession, this is something that unfortunately gets taken-for-granted. But thinking about values now, and regularly thereafter, is one important way to stay relevant and connected with our primary interest: the health and well-being of clients.

Relevant Values and Ethics to Guide Nursing Practice

- We believe in human dignity and worth
- Human beings have the right to be respected
- Human beings have the right not to be discriminated against
- All people should have equal opportunities to meet their basic human needs
- Health care should be for the well-being of the person or group
- We believe in working with and for clients, not on them

Reader Activity: Most nations now have a Code of Ethics for Nursing, which enables the profession and the public to have a transparent mechanism for accountability.
Explore the internet to find your country's code of ethics.

Nursing is about being efficient and effective, proficient in the language and techniques of medicine and science *and also* being strategic in the humane and compassionate approach taken with people during times of life transition. This is what is meant by nurses being 'transition workers' (Buchanan, 1997; Walker, 1997). Being a transition worker, means working during times of transition for people, and helping them to cross a bridge between one state (perhaps illness) into another (perhaps wellness, or adaptation). So nursing is about being able to be with clients and their family so that they transform what may be a life crisis into a turning point, something manageable. It is about giving people self-belief, resources, hope and facilitating change. It is about preventing problems as well as managing them; about helping clients as well as showing them how to help themselves. It is about noticing and responding to signs of illness as well as about imagining health broadly. It is about listening to problems as well as opening up new spaces to talk about solutions. So, next time someone asks you why do you want to be a nurse, you can answer ...

Because I want the opportunity to be able to be with people during their most significant and challenging life experiences, in ways that are supportive, helpful and needed ... Because I see nursing as an important way that I can contribute to building a happier, healthier, more connected society.

This is why this book is about solutions. It is based on the assumption that we can reorient our focus from thinking that problems are at the centre of living, towards restoring a healthy balance. Problems are part of life, just as ritual, routine, peace and happiness are. For a full and happy life to be sustained, three elements must exist in balance: health for the body; harmony for the planet; and peace for the spirit. And the focus for nursing is at three levels of change: Change in clients, change in nursing and change in society.

However, the nurse–client relationship is frequently polarized so that the nurse is the expert and the client is in receipt of care. This dualistic thinking subtly yet powerfully creates a hierarchy that digs out a trench between the nurse and client, keeping them separate and in tension.

Reader Activity: 1. Complete the missing words in this table of binary opposites.

One	The Other
Day	Night
Good	......
....	Black
Young	......
Same	Different
....	Them
Well	......
Science	......
Hard	Soft
First World	....
Whiteness	....

2. Now that the table is complete, which side represents the favoured view? What does this say about, and do to, all of the associated words?
3. Examine how each of these binary oppositions or dichotomies construct, contain and mythologise cultural understandings.
4. Make a list of other taken-for-granted, or unnoticed binary oppositions that function within health care.
5. Binary thinking can encourage people to think that differences between groups are natural, rather than cultural. Binary thinking is what helps mainstream groups to go on thinking that their values are more right than other groups. Examine characteristics of a dominant group with the group that is marginalized or oppressed.

The dominant feels	The other feels
Superior	Inferior
Dogmatic and may convey sexism/racism	Victimised
Self righteous	More violence
United	Isolated
Strong	Powerless
Alienated from one's body and nature	Group is divided
No empathy for those who are different	Helpless to change
Redemptive	Learned helplessness

Here are some important binaries that can be thought about more cautiously or even replaced.

Us/Them: This binary is dominant in health care. But nurses are not always the 'us' because depending on context, nurses actually feel like, and are positioned as 'them'. Take for example, the traditional team meeting. Many nurses have complained that their assessments are not valued or listened to. Another example is when nurses are joked about and diminished. Being treated like an object is the ultimate in being 'them' or the 'other'. Also, clients are not always the 'other', especially if they have social roles of authority, or if they become influential by way of the consumer movement. Therefore, us/them is an ill-fitting and unhelpful binary that reduces and contains nurses and clients. An alternative is to think of clients and nurses as being 'partners', where it might be possible to conceptualize them joined as 'we'. By focusing on commonalities rather than differences, we can suggest ways to work together on joint issues.

Sick/Well: This is another dominant binary that is gradually being recognized as artificial and irrelevant to contemporary health care. Public health is the agenda for the future that can be driving health services. Therefore, all health service providers need to consider potential clients as just as likely to be healthy members of the community in need of primary prevention such as health education, as they are to be sick people in need of secondary services such as treatment and rehabilitation.

The trouble with seeing the world in terms of binaries, or using predominantly dualistic thinking to assess situations, is that it usually only uncovers tension, it doesn't suggest alternatives. An approach to thinking that does help to reframe the situation is dialectical thinking.

Dialectics, is a term that was coined by Hegel, a German philosopher, and was originally used to explain the reality of tensions in all things co-existing. For example, we all have feminine as well as masculine traits, but to recognize this, one needs to engage in some conscious analysis. In what way am I feminine? In what way am I not feminine? In what way am I masculine? In what way am I not masculine? This set of questions offers a way to see both sides of an issue, to examine the thesis and anti-thesis. Since nurses are in the business of people work (and people differ along many lines, be it by gender, religion, culture or sub-culture), it is essential that we make an effort to understand both sides of issues, to appreciate complexity, to be curious about other ways to solve problems than just the conventional.

The conventional approach to problem solving involves primarily left brain thinking. One thinks about the problem, assesses it using knowledge skills, then devises a plan to solve the problem drawing on evidence, books, advice or common sense to generate alternative solutions. The solution is implemented and later effects are evaluated. This is a methodical approach often called the scientific problem-solving process.

An alternative to this is the dialectical approach. To illustrate, imagine this scenario. You've just been invited to lunch by Anne, a Director of Nursing.

She seems like a nice person, so you accept. After you both order, Anne says suddenly, 'You know there's something I've been dying to tell you about. It's a new idea I have and because you're new to clinical work, I'd really like to know what you think'.
'OK', you say 'go ahead'.
Anne goes on

> Now, I'm going to be controversial here, but I sense that you are different to most of the young students I meet, so I'm going out on a limb here. I think that access to Higher Education for nursing was a mistake. In fact I'd go so far as to say that it's possibly the worst thing that could have happened to the health care industry. No longer do health services have any control over the training that nurses receive to work in our local contexts. You know, sometimes we have specialised units that we simply cannot staff because the nurses lack the necessary skills when they graduate.

Spend a few moments playing 'the believing game' and the next few moments playing 'the doubting game'. This game involves thinking about why Anne might see things the way she does. What can you understand about her point of view? What might you agree with? Then, shift your stance and critically analyse her theory. What is she ignoring? What fault do you find with her reasoning? How does your experience offer contrary evidence?

Looking at an issue from both sides is what is meant by dialectical thinking. Moving back and forth between observations and ideas helps to deepen inquiry and appreciate complexity in issues.

Reader Activity: Analyse these issues using dialectical thinking:

1. 'Client' is the most appropriate term to use for users of the health care system.
2. Learning nursing can involve more applied science education than social science.
3. Clients are the experts of their illness and therefore, there is no place for others telling them what to do.

In the solution orientation, a conscious effort is made in removing binaries, moderating the hierarchical stance by sharing expertise, privileging the client's voice, ideas, language and goals. A deliberate attempt is made to be open, collaborative and respectful. In assessment interviews with clients, an effort is made to generate two-way conversation using inquiry and asking questions that focus on goals and strategies for change. Using a strengths perspective helps to focus on the development of potential, rather than the magnifying of limitations which can tend to be produced by concentrating on deficits

Table 3.1 Summary of the strengths model adapted from Rapp (1998)

Definition
The strengths model of assessment focuses on exploring and understanding peoples' abilities not just their disabilities.
It is concerned with, and curious about, what protects people from disorder, and what keeps them well.

Aim
It aims to assist consumers in identifying, securing and sustaining the range of resources needed to live, play, and work in a normally interdependent way in the community.

Assumptions about human behaviour
People are successful in everyday life when they use and develop their own potential And when they have access to resources needed to do this.

Protective factors
Certain protective factors exist within many individuals and groups that somehow assists them to remain well, despite facing adversity. It is useful to identify these factors in order that we can build them up in clients and ourselves.

1. Child factors: social competence, social skills, above average intelligence, attachment to family, empathy, problem-solving
2. Family factors: caring parents, harmony, more than two years between siblings, stable, small, strong family norms and morality
3. School context: positive climate, pro-social peer group, required helpfulness, sense of belonging, opportunities for success, school norms concerning violence
4. Life events: meeting significant person, moving to a new area, opportunities at critical turning points
5. Community and culture: access to support, networking, pride, identity, participation

(see Table 3.1). During the building phase of the relationship it is helpful to use strategies that help the client stay focused on reaching goals and by seeing the problem as manageable. Scaling change and externalizing questions can be useful.

The goal in the nurse–client relationship is to channel the client towards goals or desired actions. It is important in encounters with clients to try to imagine future possibilities where the problem is not so significant, to develop hopefulness. A technique that can be used is to focus on exceptions and hidden or potential resources. In encounters with clients, nurses have a role in helping them to find meaning and manageability in health problems. By focusing less on logic and reason, and more on creative thinking, nurses can use imagery, metaphors and narratives to reframe and de-centre problems and to build strengths and capacity in the client and social supports. Small signs of progress and steps towards goal achievement need to be noticed and commemorated, so that the everyday is not overlooked but scrutinized.

In my experience, I think the best nurses are those who manage to be creative in thinking, yet systematic in practice. They manage to:

- Be knowledgeable about illnesses, treatments and best practice ... yet humble and willing to learn what the client can teach them
- Be compassionate and flexible ... yet focused and disciplined about providing orderly treatments and care
- Think outside the square ... yet stay squarely on target
- Be able to speak up and out ... yet willing to do more listening that talking Being clear about these values is an important step towards being able to rethink practice and become solution focused. The next step is to develop skills in critical reflection.

Skills in Critical Reflection

Contrary to many peoples' beliefs, nursing does not come naturally to all practical, commonsense folk. In fact, you will shortly read an account of an event that happened that illustrates an astounding degree of absence of common sense. Nursing actually does need to be learned, thought about, practiced and developed. If it is to be developed then we need to think about practice critically, using the concept of 'critical reflection'. Critical reflection in Solution-Focused Nursing is a whole brain endeavour. You don't just need logic and reason to be highly developed; you also need to exercise your creative muscles.

Critical reflection aims for awareness. Two main awareness raising strategies are to clarify personal values, and to be constantly interpretive of surrounding events.

Take a look at these left- and right-brain attributes (see Table 3.2).

Many of us may agree that nurses are well known for their intuitive skills and perhaps also for their logic, but the point I'm trying to emphasize is that the skills needed for being solution-focused, are not either left or right, they are both left and right.

Table 3.2 Left- and right-brain attributes

Left hemisphere		*Right hemisphere*	
Analytic	Linear	Intuitive	Non-verbal
Logical	Verbal	Spontaneous	Imaginative
Orderly	Factual	Diffuse	Metaphoric
Systematic	Concrete	Descriptive	Abstract

(Adapted from Cherry *et al.* 1993)

Let's apply these insights to critically reflecting on the following simple, yet profound story that took place recently.

> Jenny, 38 years old, had recently returned from surgery where she had undergone a choleycystectomy. She had an IV in situ, as well as patient-controlled analgesia. Her doctor had advised her that becoming mobile as soon as possible following the procedure would facilitate recovery.
>
> Two hours post-op, Jenny was feeling the effects of a full bladder. As she made her way slowly and unsteadily to the bathroom, Jenny passed by two nurses busily talking to each other and making a bed. Fumbling to balance toiletries and also keep the IV pole untangled as she walked, Jenny dropped a hand-towel directly in front of the two nurses.
>
> Without stopping to help retrieve the fallen articles, or to assist the client to make safe passage to the bathroom, the nurses continued blithely on with the bed-making task and their private conversation.
>
> Unbeknownst to these young graduates, Jenny was an experienced nurse educator who passionately espoused the value and humanizing potential of nursing. So, aside from the pain and discomfort that went unattended, she felt disappointed by the lack of compassion shown to her, and disheartened that, after so much activity and advances in the discipline, nurses could approach their work so routinely.

Critical Reflection

This story was deliberately chosen to reflect an encounter that was unplanned, because that is how many interactions between nurses and clients operate in the everyday. When the encounter is predicted, such as during a formal assessment interview, then it is more likely that a nurse will have time to plan the approach, have explicit goals for the encounter, and consciously choose sound communication and helping skills. But in a chance encounter, as in this scenario, values about clients, nursing, work and society tend to leak out and reveal themselves. If we are not fully aware of our values, then we are less able to reflect on them and change them. These unconscious attitudes then slip out unnoticed, damaging relationships and damaging nursing.

So let's begin to deconstruct this story. To start, we need to reflect on our own values about nursing. I'm going to assume that you agree with mine. That is, that the goals for all nurse–client interactions are to provide comfort and to help the client live a happier, healthier, more connected life. Next, we need to compare our own values with what we interpret to be the values of the nurses in the story. We cannot really know what their values are without talking with them, but we can draw upon the evidence at hand – what they do, what they don't do, the perceptions that the client has of them.

Some important evidence concerning the behaviour of the two nurses is that they are focused on the task and not on the client and they are talking to each other and not with the client. They are not responsive to triggers in the environment which might require them to adapt and respond – such that they do not even notice an incapacitated, potentially unsafe client, possibly in need of assistance. They are locked in to habit and routine. And ultimately they appear to be non-reflective, non-aware.

We can all benefit from thinking about the part we play in interactions, because it helps create possibilities for improvements. When it comes to nursing practice, without an openness for self-reflection and critique, the individual as well as the profession runs the risk of becoming rigid, inflexible and irrelevant.

So, critical reflection is important for keeping nursing dynamic and responsive. At the individual level, the benefit of regular critical reflection is that it develops skills that may be weak, helps to ensure that we are responsive to the needs of others and it also means that daily work poses continual questions for us. It is challenging rather than repetitive and boring.

Reader Activity: Imagine you had just returned from theatre, you dropped something but were ignored by two nurses working directly near you. How would you feel?

Another way to interpret this encounter is to notice a problem in focus. The nurses have over-focused on being task-oriented, procedural, and left-brained. They have failed to use intuition and common sense and as a result they have been neglectful and unconscious of unintended effects. They have unwittingly allowed an us/them binary to emerge, to the extent where Jenny, the client, felt insignificant, indeed invisible. The nurses here have dismissed their own potential to think holistically and missed an opportunity to work in partnership with the client and to give her/him the power, skills and confidence to make his/her own assessment and decisions.

Reader Activity: What are the consequences for the client when a nurse takes an exclusively task focus to a situation?
What are the consequences for nursing?
Suggest an insight-raising response that Jenny could have said to make the nurses notice their behaviour.

Still another way to interpret the encounter is to look for the silences. There's another nurse in the story, who so far has not been scrutinized. Jenny, the client in the story, is also a nurse and as such also has a role to play in being solution-focused. Arguably, she too has missed an opportunity to build a connection with the two nurses, to alert them to her need and perhaps later to discuss with them her tension – of being both a client and a nurse, and the difficulties of that position. Perhaps she could have found a way to talk about being on the receiving end of care, and how disempowering that feels, or how hard it is to ask for help when usually you are in a position of authority and control. By practicing critical reflection on encounters such as these, I think that nurses can become more self-aware and more effective carers.

Now let's take a look at another interaction, this time one that proceeds along more solution-focused lines.

Working at the Interpersonal Level

Nurse: Hello Sam, remember me, I'm Jane. Thanks for talking yesterday about the surgery that is planned. We talked a lot. You showed that you have a good understanding of the actual procedure as well as the risks associated with it. We also talked about the anxious feelings you have. As we agreed yesterday, today we will be spending some time getting to know your situation more deeply, what your concerns are, as well as your goals in working together with me. How does that sound?

Sam: That sounds ok. What would you like to know?

Jane: Well, there's a lot I don't know, and I'm not the expert on you, you are. But I guess a good place to begin would be with our situation, our relationship right now. Sam, I wonder if you could tell me, what needs to come out of this meeting so that you can say this is helpful?

Sam: I don't know. Maybe to feel less anxious, to feel like I can take charge of these jangly nerves, I don't know, to feel more confident that I think I can get through this.

Jane: Ok, so it sounds like what you want is to feel more in control of the Jangly Nerves. Let's look at these Jangly Nerves in closer detail. On a scale of 1–10 (1 being least 10 being worst) how would you rate those Jangly Nerves now?

Sam: I'd say a 6.

Jane: And where on the scale would you like to be, so that you felt calm and ok.

Sam: I'd say 4 would be good.

Jane: Alright 4 would be good. And how would 5 feel?

Sam: If I could get to feeling 5 by the end of today, then that would be a great start.

Jane: Yes, I agree, it really would. So let's talk about those jangly nerves some more. Sam, when do they seem more obvious, more out there?

Sam: I have no idea. They're always there.

Jane: Well, suppose I asked your wife to answer that question. What do you think she'd say?

Sam: That's easy, she'd say it's when ever something happens that might take me away from always being in charge. She says I just hate it when things happen that I can't control.

Jane: Oh, that's interesting. So now, I wonder what your wife would say you are like when you are calmer. Do you think she'd be able to think of times when your Jangly Nerves are not so apparent.

Sam: She'd probably say I'm calm when I've had a holiday, when I'm lying in my hammock reading a detective story. As a matter of fact those are some times when I'm quite ok.

Jane: So, suppose a miracle happened over night, and the jangly nerves just went away. What would you be doing and feeling, can you describe that to me?

Sam: I'd be cool, calm, collected, able to go into that surgery knowing that I was doing the right thing, and pretty much accepting of the surgeon's skills.

Jane: Maybe if we tried using some of the cool, calmness that seems to come out when you're lying in that hammock, and applying it to this situation, your jangly nerves might be less obvious. What do you think?

Sam: Well, I'm willing to give it a try ...

For some people, being solution-oriented instead of problem focused is like learning a new language. It can be quite stilted and frustrating at first. It takes practice to talk with people differently about their health status, and conditions.

Furthermore, there is more than one way to approach encounters such as this one. Jane could have begun the conversation much less directly, and more creatively. Go to the list of further readings, if you would like to find out more on this topic.

If you look back on the encounter you will see a number of question techniques that are aiming to help the client notice and talk about their strengths and not just their vulnerabilities or needs. You will also find questions and comments that aim to build up hope in the client, to convey a sense of optimism, that the problem can be contained and managed.

The following section provides suggestions adapted from Insoo Kim Berg and Peter de Jong, leading solution-focused counselors, to help you feel comfortable in crafting similar solution-building conversations.

Focus on asking 'Wh' Questions (What, Who, Where, When, Which, and How)

- What needs to come out of this meeting so that you can say this is helpful?
- What tells you that you are at 5?
- Tell me about the times when you are more productive? What is different then?
- How would that be helpful to you?
- What has been changed, even a little bit, since you made this appointment?

Use Collaborative Language

- Be tentative, rather than forthright because the former style is more humble and collaborative. The latter style is typical of the expert, who always has the answers. A forthright style can be silencing. It can encourage the person to feel stupid or unskilled. For example, use words like 'maybe', 'suppose', 'it appears', 'it sounds like' and check out your perceptions with the client.
- Use the person's own words to describe their experiences.
- Show agreement, enthusiasm, support and optimism. These feelings may be contagious and the client may begin to share them and feel more confident about resolving their situation.

Ask Building Questions

- Questions like 'What would your best friend (boss, mother) say you are like when you are calmer?' help to put the problem into an external space, where they can be noticed and analysed more impartially. This is a kind of externalizing question. Another way to use externalizing language is to help the person see the problem as something separate, and therefore not forever linked, to them as a person. Calling the problem 'the jangly nerves' makes it objectified, and more easily manipulated out of the person's life.
- Questions like 'Can you think of a time when the jangly nerves were less prominent?' is a way to help the person search for exceptions to their problem-focus. It's tempting to always engage in trouble-talk, and when we do, it isn't long before we start thinking about our whole life as beset with problems and illness. Finding exceptions to the illness stories, makes a space for optimism and change.
- Change oriented questions are a focus for nurse-client work, and scaling questions are often useful. For example, 'On a scale of 1–10, how would you rate your nerves' is helpful in establishing a base line, and then to move towards small steps for change. Asking 'what would we need to do to move you one increment closer to calm?' and 'How close to your goals have your moved so far?' and 'What is the next small step you need to take toward your goal?' are all useful in keeping the change moving.
- Miracle questions enable the person to be able to imagine a different scenario to the one that is presently so troubling, but it's often really hard to picture when you feel rotten, in pain, or upset. For example, 'What if a miracle happened and the problem went away. What would you be doing differently?, Paired with a scaling question like 'What is the first small thing that could change' starts to thicken up the image so that the person can actually see what the change will look like.

So now we have explored one of three foci for solution focused nursing: working with clients at the interpersonal level. As we know, being solution focused also requires nurses to be involved at the social level, working collaboratively with other nurses to build connections and community so that change in nursing itself is produced.

Working at the Social Level

Even though there's a lot of potential in nursing – health care work is extremely important to a community's well-being, there are many making huge contributions to society – there are also many challenges. Nurses have been described as an oppressed group that often feels undervalued, misunderstood, silenced and marginalized (Roberts, 1983). It suffers from over-active self-criticism, disunity and power struggles. It is preoccupied with its own identity and goals. Understanding this concept of oppression helps to explain why some nurses are hostile, competitive or critical of other nurses. But it can also point to solutions (Skelton, 1993).

There are many stories of oppressed groups that have managed to overcome adverse conditions and become empowered. Sometimes in looking at their experiences, we can begin to find new ways of looking at our own. Using stories to reveal lessons about the self is another example of using the externalizing strategy explored in the previous section. The Yackandandah community of Victoria has one such story that I think has lessons for nursing (Vichealth, 2004).

Singing Amidst the Ashes

In the early part of this decade, Australia's south east was ravaged by fire. Many people lost their homes and livelihoods. It was a sad and desperate time, especially for the people of Yackandandah, in Victoria. But some irrepressible members of the community came up with the idea that singing might help the process of recovery. With some government funding, the local choir organized singing workshops. The aim was simply to bring people together, take their minds off their own personal troubles and do something positive for the group.

Soon, there was an opportunity to join a theatre company to tour other isolated communities, bringing music and stories of hope. 'We believe in the power of music in all its different forms, to connect people, to lift people's spirits and to take people's minds off their troubles,' said a local participant at the time. 'It is very hard to think of how bad things are when you're singing!'

I'm not suggesting that nurses all start singing operettas, but I do think there are some insights here. There is value in people coming together around a common cause. It can take the focus away from differences and people can learn that they share more than they differ. The story also shows that it can help to limit trouble talk and worrying about the past, by focussing on the future. It can be motivating and unifying when groups focus less on themselves and more on the needs of others.

So the moral of this story for you is that there will be situations in your future professional practice that make you feel proud to be part of the discipline of nursing, but there will also be times when you feel isolated and unsupported. The challenge for you will be in transforming these difficult moments into turning points.

Reader Activity: Nurses have a tendency not to call attention to achievements or publicly validate each other. In order to give you an opportunity to be different, here's a challenge for when you are next visiting a clinical agency.
Observe and document an effective nurse–nurse interaction. It might be a senior colleague offering praise to a junior nurse. It might be a gentle way of communicating a critique of performance. In what way did it contrast from what is normally done in similar circumstances?
What was it that was actually said?
What was it about the tone of the interaction that impressed you?
Approach the colleague, and let them know what, how and why you were so impressed.
Notice the effect that this disclosure has on the individual and on you.

Working at the Cultural Level

Another important focus for nursing is at the cultural level. Even though many people probably think of nursing as a role that is focused primarily at the individual level – helping clients and families cope with ill-health, or perhaps working in schools to promote well-being and healthy lifestyles, nursing has long been concerned with and active in, the social world. When working at the cultural level particular skills are useful to develop (Allan, 2003). These include:

Advocacy	Mediating and interceding for clients, only when the client seeks representation, and in an attempt to influence the behaviours of decision-makers.
Capacity building	Creating an enabling environment that empowers clinicians, carers and communities to engage in sustainable community development; providing staff and carer support, education, links and networks.
Activating groups	Facilitating change-oriented groups to link people in so that they can enjoy the positive effects of being part of a group, develop an outward, future-orientation, and influence decision makers themselves.
Public communication	Presenting at consumer, professional and national levels to disseminate insights from research, advance the discourse for clients and nurses, challenge conventional thinking and develop alliances.
Elegant challenging	Questioning the actions and attitudes of others in tactful and constructive ways that allow people to save face and that avoid unnecessary hostilities and tensions.

To me, Florence Nightingale illustrates all that I have tried to emphasize about solution-focused work at the interpersonal, social and cultural levels. She embodied and linked compassion with discipline and hard work. She was active at the individual level, providing comfort and care to soldiers in the Crimean war. She was a leader at the social level, educating nurses and health care workers, providing structures, protocols, rules and procedures to increase effectiveness and efficiency. And as you can see from the letter below, she was active at the cultural level, making an effort to influence policy and politicians on matters to do with health and social well-being.

Read the following letter from Florence Nightingale sent to the Manchester Guardian Newspaper over 100 years ago. Consider the cultural skills present in the piece and analyse its meaning for contemporary nursing.

Miss Florence Nightingale has sent a letter to Mr Alex Devine, of the Goden Boy's Home and the Mission to Lads at the Police Courts, Manchester, on the subject of the treatment of juvenile offenders. Miss Nightingale writes:

> *the work you are doing at Manchester in rescuing boys 'had up' for their first offence is one of overhwhelming importance, and yours is, as far as I know, the first and only one of its kind ... It is astounding that a practical nation like the English should have done so little (about this). We have a vague idea that 75 per cent of the boys committed to our reformatories are reformed and do well. We have a vague idea that 75 per cent of those committed to gaol return there again and again. ... it (is) a complete non sequitur that because a boy stole your watch he should be supported on your rates in gaol, perhaps for life, and suggested that he might be made to work out the price of what he stole ... It would be of immense importance if the public had kept before them the statistics, well worked out, of the influence of punishment on crime or reformatories and industrial schools on juvenile offenders. It has been truly said that 'criminology' is much less studied than 'insectology' ... Another subject of statistical research is, Do paupers and the children of paupers return again and again to the workhouse? And in what proportion do the same names appear generation after generation on the books? I could write much more, but I have no power of following up the subject. For the last 40 years I have been immersed in two objects and have undertaken what might well occupy 20 vigorous young people, and I am an old and overworked invalid. God bless you, and bless your work and multiply it a thousand-fold.*

Excerpt from: Bettman/Corbis. (2004). From the archives: Dealing with young offenders, from the Manchester Guardian, 5 September 1890. The Guardian Review, 9 October 2004. p. 24.

Reader Activity: Discuss the surface level reading of this story and its relevance today.

Appraise the cultural helping skills evident within.

Think about the subject under discussion. Is this a public conversation to which you hear many nurses contributing? What does this say about Nightingale?

Explore and highlight any hidden binaries.
Suggest a dialectical reading.
What attributes of Nightingale are relevant and irrelevant to today's conceptions of nursing?
To what extent are nurses visible in the public spheres, such as in politics and social welfare?

Conclusion

Doing nursing differently requires vision, commitment and new skills. Like any change, if this different way of nursing is to take hold, then individuals and groups must see the need, believe in the way forward and have the motivation to get moving.

By now, the concept of Solution-Focused Nursing ought to be becoming more clear. Whilst underpinned by some complex notions about society, knowledge and change, perhaps it can be boiled down to 6 key principles. These are:

1. The person, not the problem, is at the centre of inquiry.
2. Problems and strengths may be present at all times. Looking for and then developing inner strengths and resources will be affirming and assist in coping and adaptation. By working with what's going right with a client, one can be enhancing their hope, optimism and self-belief, thus maximizing their health capacity.
3. Resilience is as important as vulnerability.
4. The nurse's role moves beyond illness-care towards adaptation and recovery.
5. The goal is to create change at 3 levels: in the client, nursing and society. Thus it requires nurses to go beyond individual-focused care, to valuing the role of social and cultural care. It involves noticing practices that might be unhelpful or unjust and aiming to instead put in place empowering, enabling strategies. Understanding is not sufficient to enact change, one must be active, involved and committed.
6. The way of being with clients is proactive, rather than reactive. Care involves three phases of joining – or getting to know the person rather than the diagnosis; building, developing skills and resources the client can use to recover and adapt; and extending, opportunity for the client to practice these new skills and to connect with further social supports

In this chapter we have focused on the groundwork that is necessary so that new skills will sink in, be remembered, embraced and used. We have explored:

- Critical thinking and reflection on practice
- The importance of noticing taken-for-granted beliefs/practices

- The role of surfacing personal values in order to shape practice
- Binaries and the place for dialectical thinking
- Solution-building questions
- Community building stories that provide life lessons for nurses working with and for each other
- Our role and responsibility for making change at the cultural level.

Suggestions for Further Reading

McAllister, M., and Walsh, K. (2004). Different voices: Reviewing and revising the politics of working with consumers in mental health. *International Journal of Mental Health Nursing, 13*(1), 22–32.

Thompson, N. (1998). *Promoting equality: Challenging discrimination and oppression in the human services.* London: Macmillan.

Walsh, K., McAllister, M., and Morgan, A. (2002). Using reflective practice processes to identify practice change issues in an aged care service. *Nurse Education in Practice*; 2:230–236.

References

Allan, J. (2003). Practising critical social work. In, J. Allen, B. Pease and L. Briskman (eds), *Critical social work: An introduction to theories and practices.* (pp. 52–72). Crows Nest, NSW: Allen and Unwin.

Berg, I., and de Jong, P. (1998). *Interviewing for solutions.* Pacific Grove, CA: Brooks/Cole.

Bettman/Corbis. (2004). From the archives: Dealing with young offenders, from the Manchester Guardian, 5 September 1890. *The Guardian Review*, 9 October 2004. p. 24.

Buchanan, T. (1997). Nursing our narratives: Towards a dynamic understanding of nurses in narrative tales. *Nursing Inquiry, 4*, 80–87.

Cherry, C., Godwin, D., and Staples, J. (1993). *Is the left brain always right?* Melbourne: Hawker Brownlow Education.

Rapp, C. (1998). *The strengths model: Case management with people suffering severe and persistent mental illness.* New York: Oxford University Press.

Roberts, S. (1983). Oppressed group behaviour: Implications for nursing. *Advances in Nursing Science, 5*(4), 21–30.

Skelton, R. (1994). Nursing and empowerment: Concepts and strategies. *Journal of Advanced Nursing, 19*, 415–423.

VicHealth (2004). Together we do better campaign. Accessed on the internet at www.togetherwedobetter, 23 October, 2004.

Walker, K. (1997). Dangerous liaisons: Thinking, doing, nursing. *Collegian, 4*(2), 4–6, 8–14.

CHAPTER 4

Families in Transition: Early Parenting

Jennifer Rowe and Margaret Barnes

Overview

This chapter is about families, specifically families undergoing change and transition as a result of childbearing. The family is a rich, diverse and dynamic entity, and a crucial societal building block. Its good functioning is important for establishing and sustaining many psycho-social dimensions of life. The advent of a baby, while welcomed in most families, is challenging, particularly for parents. This is regardless of whether they have prior parenting experience, or are facing parenting for the first time. The intention in this chapter is to focus on the parents as key people in family transition. A number of situations are discussed in which nurses can engage creatively and helpfully with parents. First, three short stories or snapshots are presented. Background and foundational knowledge about family and parenting transition is provided, before the reader is taken into the various nursing contexts to consider and apply principles of supportive and enabling practice.

Stories

Marika and Stefan

It is 1.20pm and Marika, 32, is sitting by the humidicrib in the neonatal intensive care nursery. Marika arrived at seven this morning. It is two weeks since her little girl was born, six weeks before her due date. The room is filled with alarms, voices and shuffling. Doctors and nurses surround the crib in the next bay. Marika is watching her baby startle in response to an alarm from another crib. She leans over the crib and places her hands into the portal to gently stroke her baby. Her thoughts turn to the coming weekend. She hasn't had a chance to do any shopping and her partner Stefan has organised to have his children for the weekend.

Bruce and Patanee

Bruce and Patanee are planning a day in town, over an hour away from their home. While they are in town they plan to visit the child health service. Their first baby, Jack, is now five months old, fully breastfed and doing well. They plan to ask the nurse about starting the baby on solid foods, prompted in part by Bruce's mother's recent comments about the baby soon needing something more than milk. Also, Patanee has been reading a few pamphlets and parenting guides which seem to say different things. She has discussed this during phone conversations with her mother, a Thai national living in Thailand. Her mother's views are traditional; she is concerned about the quality of Patanee's milk and worries that if Patanee doesn't feed Jack for long enough he will be stubborn. During the conversation with the nurse at the clinic, Bruce comments that he doesn't feel very involved yet but guesses this will come when Jack is older.

Joanne

Joanne is 17 and pregnant for the first time. At her recent antenatal visit at the hospital Joanne met a community health nurse who works as part of a post birth home visiting service. The nurse has encouraged Joanne to join the service. Joanne came away feeling that she doesn't have much choice. However, she rings the nurse and agrees to take part, organising a meeting for the following week.

Foundations

The men and women in these stories are in transition. Their sense of self, responsibilities and lifestyle are changing because of the advent of a baby in their lives; an utterly dependent, vulnerable and challenging being who requires complete care. For each, the well-being of the infant, then toddler, young child and adolescent will depend, in part, on her/his beginning care, interactions and relationships. They are also families in transition. These transitions are not only foundational for individual personhood, but also for families and for the communities of the future. In the contemporary world, the importance of links between family, parenting and childhood health and well-being are well recognized and form the focus of significant government and non government attention around the globe. They are written into policies, resourced in health and community care services, supplied in a range of private enterprise endeavours, and supported and facilitated in everyday encounters with friends, family and health professionals, such as nurses.

The stories evoke images of very different families. The contemporary family in Australia, the United Kingdom, North America and many other developed nations may be characterised in the following comments by Saggers and Sims (2005). Speaking of the Australian context they compare the historical normality of the nuclear family, of mum, dad and kids with today's families:

> the realities of sole-parent families, step- and blended families, extended families, same-sex families, childless households, and even the single person household where the strongest ties are not with biological kin but with intimate friends. Add to this the diversity of ethnic and cultural backgrounds that Indigenous Australians and postwar migrating families contribute and all Australians will eventually encounter family types quite different to their own. (Saggers and Sims, 2005, p. 66)

The principles are common to all these societies no matter what the specific details of history and politics in each. What is important is the significance of diversity and difference. Diversity and difference are important concepts not only to understand theoretically but to also operationalise, when as health professionals, nurses consider the strengths, opportunities and aspirations of the families they support. Add to this two other concepts resulting from the birth of a child, transition and change, and the complexity of practice becomes evident. But so too, the privilege of working with one of the engine rooms of society, the family, generates a sense of challenge and excitement.

Reader Activity: Conduct an on-line internet search of your national and provincial or state government websites for policy in relation of parenting and families. What part of government is focused on this area? What needs and strengths are identified? What services are promoted to respond to needs?

The meaning a family gives to the birth of a child will, in part, construct the way family members, particularly parents, assess and perceive the event. In turn this construction and meaning may influence personal and family dynamics – the way a family feels and acts (McKenry and Price, 2000). Important to these family dynamics and the way a family will function in the face of them, are resources. Resources are defined as abilities or characteristics of individuals, families and communities that meet the demands associated with changes and transitions (McCubbin and Patterson, 1985). Personal resources include self-esteem and good physical health. Adequate financial resources help a family, and finally, good community health and human services on which family members may call, are also resources. Embedded in each parent's resources are ideals and expectations, hopes and aspirations, worries and concerns – for themself, the other members of their family and their young child.

Parenting, Identity and Nurturing Roles

For both women and men, parenting is multifaceted and dynamic. All parents, but in particular first time parents, face new challenges and disruptions as they realize the impact a new baby has on their lives (Nyström and Öhrling, 2004). At the heart of transition to mothering and fathering are issues of identity and nurturing work (Barclay and Lupton, 1999; Hays, 1996; Rane and McBride, 2000; Rogan, Schmied, Barclay, Everitt, and Wylie, 1997).

Take mothers and mothering first. For women, the period of transition into new motherhood has been described as a developmental process and given time, opportunity and experience, women acquire the skills and confidence to successfully adapt to or incorporate this role (Barclay *et al.*, 1997). However, while this transition is part of a developmental process, many find it a difficult period in their lives (Nyström and Öhrling, 2004). In addition, historically, families have played a key role in meeting women's needs. It is still common practice in many parts of the world for women to learn about birth and baby care from their own mothers, sisters and other female relatives (Nolan, 1997). In contemporary, developed nations, however, there is recognition and concern that new mothers are often socially and geographically isolated from their family and friends. Many women have been raised in a small nuclear family with little or no contact with new babies, thereby limiting their learning opportunities for mothering knowledge and skills, thus indicating an important role for health professional support at this time.

For women such as Marika, Patanee and Joanne, the nurturing work of mothering, that is, carrying out the everyday realities of caring for their vulnerable and dependent children, is characterised in developed countries at least, as intensive, self sacrificing, and exclusive (Arendell, 2000; Hays, 1996). The inference here is that not only will many women begin mothering with little concrete experience, in situations where they are isolated from family and friends but that high societal expectations of the quality of their mothering will shadow their efforts. However, they are not without insight. They bring to mothering various experiences, beliefs, ideas and values. They will engage with their infants in an intense, bodily relationship, characterised by dialectical tensions of nurturing the child while preserving self (Rowe, 2003), and in a balancing act in which they must facilitate the gradual individuation of baby as body and person, from themselves (Bowden, 1997).

While custom may determine the character of many of their activities mothering also carries expectations, boundaries and negotiation between the private and public, self and other. Mothers will define themselves and be defined by the way they care for their babies, but also by the way they engage their family and household, as well as other roles outside the home (Saggers and Sims, 2005; Arendell, 2000). The small decisions and actions of everyday life, therefore, do more than nurture a baby; they define and shape personhood. Supporting Joanne to understand what she brings to her new role, and how she can gather the best support possible around her from extended family as she mothers her newborn may not only help her nurture her baby well but also nurture her opportunities as a young adult. Given such important outcomes, the need for quality support in professional practice, is obvious.

Men too, face new challenges and bring experiences and expectations to fathering. Fatherhood has only recently come into focus as an important concern in scholarship and practice. Changes in societal understandings of fatherhood in the last two to three decades have resulted in ambiguous expectations about men's fathering identity and their involvement in nurturing, caregiving, activities. These have occurred in part because of changes in family life (Marsiglio, Amato, Day and Lamb, 2000), as well as shifts in wage-work dynamics and how these interact with private household work for both men and women (Dowd, 2000; Kaila-Behm and Vehviläinen-Julkunen, 2000). These dynamics are at times competing, and influence constructions of fatherhood for communities, families and individual men. The ambiguity of transition to fatherhood, as well as the nature of contemporary fatherhood, contrasts with the more clearly defined structures and dynamics of motherhood (although these constructs should not be taken as uncontested or complete) (Draper, 2003). A father such as Bruce may be uncertain of his responsibility or what to do as he begins fathering (Singleton, 2005). Does he, for example, consider himself as a bystander, supporter, head of family or partner (Kaila-Behm and Vehviläinen-Julkunen, 2000)? Fathers like Stefan may be more involved with their infants at the outset than those like Bruce, a situation born of necessity with a critically ill infant.

Men's involvement and understanding of fathering will develop over time, influenced by many factors, not least by the expectations and values of their partners (Dowd, 2000). Transition toward fatherhood is also, according to Draper (2003, p. 69), 'accomplished in relation to his partner's transition to motherhood, his parents' transition to grandparenthood, the couple's transition into a family and existing children's transition to brother or sister.' Transition for men, as for women, into parenting is thus collective as well as individual. Does Marika, for example, see Stefan as a primary caregiver for the children or a helper? Knowing may help her to cope with the stress of mothering a child in neonatal intensive care as well as her other commitments. Does Patanee see herself, or Bruce, as the decision maker or do they share decision making equally? How do Bruce and Patanee's parents' experiences and socio-cultural environments shape their transitions as individuals, and as a family?

These possibilities, tensions and issues underpin parenting realities. Solution focused nursing in the context of family transition through childbearing will concentrate much of its attention on parents. Nursing will acknowledge the abilities of parents to successfully manage the transition to parenthood, changes in the family, and the potential they have to master the tasks required. Focus will be specifically on the resources and strengths they bring as individuals, families, and in the context of their communities, as well as upon everyday, often small, things that illustrate, or make transparent, these resources. Nursing action will centre on providing support so that parents may value their hopes, identities and nurturing roles, value their families and enhance them as safe, supportive environments, and thus, provide children with the best start possible.

Contexts of Care

The context of care and support for new parents is diverse, within a range of acute and community contexts. For Marika, for example, it is the intensity of the neonatal unit. Technology in this context is important to meet an infant's treatment needs, but it is also intrusive and stressful. The challenge for care in this environment is to balance the physical needs of the baby with the psychosocial needs of the family. In this environment nursing care may focus on the needs of the baby, but equally concern and care needs to be directed to the development of the family.

The role of community health services is highlighted as well. For Bruce and Patanee it is the child health service in a rural township and for Joanne, the offer of a home visiting service. The role of community nursing services in providing support for new families is well recognized (Rowe and Barnes, in press; Barnes, Courtney, Pratt and Walsh, 2003; Fagerskiold and Ek, 2003), however, services differ across geographical contexts and the extent to which they are provided universally, or for targeted populations, varies.

The role of the nurse in these situations, and others, may be one of caregiver, but it will certainly be one of supporter, counsellor, health promoter and resource person (Barnes, Courtney, Pratt and Walsh, 2004). The role has a facilitative focus and as such is well suited to solution focused approaches.

Nursing Responses

Whatever the context, interactions that are supportive, and capacity building will be at the heart of solution focused nursing responses in situations such as those described in this chapter's stories. One of the central ideas in solution focused nursing or therapy is that of goal setting with clients. The process needs to be collaborative and focus on things that have value or import to the parent. The focus for this process may be on parenting that achieves a good or cohesive sense of self, good family function, and with the motivation to nurture an infant or young child, look after self and others in one's family and everyday life, using resources which are sufficient, available and accessible. Assessing these qualities of parenting and family transition, helping the client to seek opportunities and re-frame or re-interpret experiences, and assessing progress are all essential elements of effective nursing responses, whether in a single encounter or through multiple interactions.

Support

Support helps to meet people's needs, or rather it helps people to be enabled to meet their own needs, as they identify, prioritize and integrate them into their everyday lives. Forms of support are many but those that have received most focus include informational, tangible and emotional. In fact it is thought that support involves and serves more than any one of these purposes in a given situation (Heath, 2004). Thus, understanding support types is important as key instruments in nursing interactions with people such as those in this chapter's stories.

Informational support holds a strong place in early parenting education and has done so in recent decades. This focus has resulted from increased public policy and health services attention to human development, bettering the progress of children and the changing societal expectations of parents and parenting (Heath, 2004). House (1981) theorised informational support as the provision of information that helps the person cope with problems; both personal and ones within their social environment. Two characteristics of information are crucial; accuracy and relevance.

Attachment to, and relationship with others, is a foundational human need, one that is established in the continuity of relationship between and infant and her/his adult carers, most usually mother (Bowden, 1997). For infants, continuity in these relationships are thought to facilitate their independence and autonomy over time. Actions and interactions that lead people to believe that they are valued and cared about are ones that may then allow a person to express and confide important issues and feelings. This is the foundation of emotional support (Heath, 2004; House, 1981).

Tangible support, also known as caregiving or instrumental support, involves concrete actions to provide physical assistance, material resources, household help to name but a few. To be effective, it must be both helpful and useful. Competent nurse caregiving is one type of tangible support, as is the facilitation of a new mother's group. Babysitting and housework assistance are two others.

Having outlined the principle characteristic of each form of support it is now possible to consider how they might be applied in nursing practice, to the situations suggested in each of the stories.

An Acute Care Setting – Marika

Marika is attempting to establish mothering attachment and care for her new baby in conditions which are well recognized as stressful and which potentially impede this process (Higgins and Dallow, 2003; Holditch-Davis and Miles, 1997; Miles, Funk and Kasper, 1992). Marika is likely to spend long hours at the crib watching and learning about her new baby, developing expertize or knowledge of her baby. It will be knowledge that intersects with that of the nurses and other health professionals, but which is also different, and will be expressed differently (Rowe, Gardner and Gardner, 2005).

Marika also has multiple other commitments to attend to, outside the nursery. As the result of having a hospitalized, preterm, baby, Marika and her partner Stefan, face a significant challenge, to not only make a successful parenting transition but to maintain family relationships and functions. Effective early parenting is important for good infant care, parent-child relationships and family function in the longer term (Doucette and Pinelli, 2004; Singer *et al.*, 1999).

Stress that affects parenting behaviour over time, such as that created by having a hospitalized, preterm baby, is also associated with impacts on a child's development and health (Deater-Deckard, 2004). This is particularly so if the child has serious or lasting health issues or disabilities or where there are few family resources and support (Cronin *et al.*, 1995; Doucette and Pinelli, 2004).

The challenge for the nurse is to help Marika to see, and accept as valuable, important, mothering, the attachment she feels and the caregiving she is able to do. It is important to focus on the small steps that facilitate her mothering and the resources she has and can draw on to mother her fragile infant. The literature suggests that mothers who believe that they have some sense of control have been shown to cope better than those who do not (Feldman-Reichman, 2000). In this situation this may be achieved through a combination of information and emotional support strategies. These will need to be enacted at the bedside, for example, by asking the woman what she is noticing about her baby, what is her best story about the baby for the morning, what features about her baby she likes, how the baby feels and responds to her touch. These stories and responses can be used as a starting point to provide information about the baby's reactions, physiology, appropriate stimulation and touch. This approach draws on the woman's insights and experiences of her infant as the basis of building understanding about the infant's health status, treatments and cares. Her stories and observations also provide a way of finding out what Marika's hopes and fears are regarding her baby, what she finds stressful. And so her personal resources can be recognised, acknowledged and built upon.

It is clear that mothers of preterm infants feel better about their parenting if they can engage in direct caregiving (Jackson, Ternestedt and Scholin, 2003). Thus, getting Marika to help as a care partner, even with small technical adjustments and treatments, and encouraging her involvement with whatever tactile cares are possible, will provide effective emotional support even when the opportunities to hold and care for the baby, as a mother, are severely limited.

Partnership and family focus are important and yet challenging for nurses in neonatal nurseries. Seeking and valuing the parent's insights and understandings, and building on these as an integral part of care planning, decision making and caregiving, will be enabling for parents in this situation. Demonstrating competent nursing care of the baby, which in turn may make parents like Marika feel that they are able to leave the bedside and go and attend to the other aspects of their life (Rowe, Gardner and Gardner, 2005) may be effective tangible support.

Child Health in the Community – Bruce and Patanee

Community child health and public health nursing services have been part of the health care landscape from the early twentieth century in a number of countries such as the United Kingdom and Australia. Traditionally, these services were dedicated to health screening and surveillance. Over time the psycho-social development and progress of infants and young children has become part of the service. Today such services continue to play a role in transitional care, incorporating parenting programs, to support parents during early childrearing (Rowe and Barnes, 2006; Barnes *et al.*, 2003). Bruce and Patanee's visit to a child health clinic is an opportunity for the nurse to provide informational support but also to help them affirm their parenting roles, thus providing emotional support.

Bruce and Patanee have all sorts of information about feeding their baby, however helping them to sift through their resources for accuracy and relevance to their lifestyle, represents informational support that might enable them. The nurse would need to find out more about what they know and value. So for example, the nurse might ask questions about what they know other parents have done, what they have read, what they think about suggestions they have heard, what they would like to do and what information they would find helpful so they can plan the introduction of food other than breastmilk.

Another nursing focus with this couple and their infant might be in helping Bruce affirm his fathering role. One of the important solution focused nursing strategies is listening and appreciating stories and encouraging clients to express their ideals and hopes. In this case the nurse could encourage Bruce to share his thoughts and experiences; what he enjoys about his baby, what he likes doing as a parent. The nurse could ask Bruce to describe his family now, perhaps even using drawings to help. Bruce could then be asked to describe the way he would like to see himself and his family in 12 months time when his child is a toddler. Bruce and the nurse could explore similarities and differences in these descriptions, speculate on skills and actions that Bruce can draw on to affirm his paternal transition and continue to enjoy and build on family life. These skills and actions and behaviours do not need to be big things, for example they might explore his skill as story teller, organiser or cook.

Reader Activity: Sit down with a piece of paper. Create a map of your family as it is today. Draw a second map of your family as you recall it from your childhood. Try to include indications of the context, members, relationships, strengths and tensions as you remember them.

Consider how other members of your family would recall family life during your childhood. Maybe you could ask them. If you do have a conversation, see if you can identify strengths, resources, motivations that may have shaped family dynamics.

A final point that is raised in Bruce and Patanee's story is that of generational and cultural influences on parenting practices. Both are important contextual sources of knowledge and influence for parents, although not givens. It is likely that Bruce's Anglo mother's parenting experience would have been at a time when parents were encouraged to introduce infants to solid foods from just a couple of months of age. Many more of Bruce's mother's generation would have formula feed their infants rather than breastfed, and milk feeding was organised around schedules. These experiences are likely to influence her beliefs about good caregiving and so, potentially will shape her conversations with her son and daughter-in-law. This approach may be fine for the younger parents and if so this would present an interesting situation for the nurse because such an approach would fall outside current accepted expert wisdom and much lay wisdom. Thai cultural influences are likely to give Patanee a positive view of breastfeeding and breastfeeding over the first year at least. Nutritional and moral issues of bonding and the child's personality are quite likely to be integral to the way she values breastfeeding (Rice and Naksook, 2001).

Transitions for Young Parents – Joanne

Regardless of age, the transition to motherhood can be a challenge (McVeigh and Smith, 2000) and many women feel unprepared. As parenting is difficult under the best of circumstances, it may be increasingly difficult for a woman having a baby during her teenage years. For Joanne, her attendance at antenatal clinic demonstrates a commitment to accessing health care for herself and her baby.

Teenage pregnancy is considered to be an at risk situation, with many young women experiencing adverse pregnancy outcomes. This premature move into motherhood may have adverse social, educational and financial effects (Brooks-Gunn and Chase-Lansdale 1991), however, SmithBattle (2003) argues that pregnancy for many teens is not seen as the devastating event, but rather part of a life course. SmithBattle (2003) describes the stigmatization often experienced by young pregnant women and discusses the way in which accepted social norms (that of older parenthood etc.) can influence the way in which teenagers are cared for. 'Clinicians treat mothers as passive, voiceless recipients rather than as active subjects whose concerns, priorities, and practices accurately reflect the imperatives and contradictions of the family and social worlds they inhabit' (2003, p. 371).

Suggesting to Joanne that she joins the home visiting programme may be seen as a helpful approach to managing a possibly 'at risk' situation. However, Joanne is not sure about the program and may have adequate supports within her family and friendship group. An alternative approach would be to ask Joanne questions which would enable her to reach her own conclusions and to recognize that she functions within her particular social world with particular needs and desires. This approach effectively provides emotional support by focussing on Joanne as an autonomous individual, capable of making choices.

A solution-focused approach to this situation may centre around what Joanne has in mind for her pregnancy and early mothering, by asking questions such as: How do you see your life after the baby is born? What sort of help do you expect you will need? Do you think it will be easy to get help when you need it? How will you know that you are doing well as a parent? These sorts of questions provide the environment for Joanne to identify her strengths and resources while ensuring that she is an active partner in her care.

A Summary for a Solution-focused Approach to Nursing with Families and Parents in Transition

The situations people and needs of families in transition are extremely diverse. However, the material set out in the previous sections shows some common underpinnings, which inform a solution focused approach to nursing in situations such as these. The following list identifies some of the priorities for a nurse working with families in transition. There are tips for action and reflection on the part of the nurse.

- First, assess the situation. Is the immediate issue indicative of a specific need for new knowledge, affirmation, or caregiving help?
- Put aside your assumptions of what is a priority, or a correct way to go about parenting.
- Be curious and interested in the parents, children, infants and other family members.
- Find out what is going well for the parent. How does the parent judge success?
- Encourage storytelling, for example small stories about what the parent is doing, how she/he feels, ask for illustrations of things that are going well. Many beliefs are embedded in people's stories and stories provide rich material for questioning and opportunities for re-interpreting and seeking solutions.
- Assess the resources the parent may be able to draw on – help them to work out how to draw on those resources and identify others that may be available and potentially useful.
- Use positive feedback and compliments which are affirming.
- Consider closely; are issues raised by parents about caregiving/nurturing, about their identity as parents or about other aspects of their lifestyle?
- Help the parent to be forward looking to reinterpret the present with the future in mind – even when this may be the next day or the next week. Ask questions that signpost or construct signposts of vision and success. The focus is on realistic goals and small steps using things that will work for the person.
- Make plans with the person.
- Assess progress – adaptation, motivation, tasks achieved, resources working.

Group Activity:

1. Discussion: In a group share and discuss the best story your parent tells about you when you were a baby. This activity puts you in the place of clients, of telling stories about personal events, people and feelings.

2. Values clarification and representations of the family: Agree that each member of the group will watch an hour of commercial television between 5 and 8 pm for 2 or 3 nights in the next week. The goal is to look at the representation of family on the advertisements. Make notes and then discuss and compare your findings with the other group members. What did you learn about media representations of the family? How do these reflect your knowledge of the family? How do these reflect your experience of family?

In a second activity you can work in pairs – you will need a large piece of paper and a number of different coloured pens/markers. Each person is to develop a family map. The map needs to focus on showing people and dynamics in regard to relational closeness and distance, aspects of decision making, household work, work outside the home, caregiving work. Interview another person in your group about their map. Consider the questions you ask – which ones work and for what reasons?

3. Developing questions: Take each story presented at the beginning of this chapter. For each one develop two key questions, one based on curiosity and one on planning for a future meeting.

Suggestions for Further Reading

Asen, E., Tomson, D., Young V., and Tomson, P. (2004). *Ten minutes for the family. Systematic interventions in primary care.* London: Routledge.

Poole, M. (ed). (2005). *Family: Changing families, changing times.* Melbourne: Allen and Unwin.

References

Arendell, T. (2000). Conceiving and investigating motherhood: The decade's scholarship. *Journal of Marriage and the Family, 62*, 1192–1207.

Barclay, L., and Lupton, D. (1999). The experience of new fatherhood: a socio-cultural analysis. *Journal of Advanced Nursing, 29*(4), 1013–1020.

Barclay, L., Everitt, L., Rogan, F., Schmied, V., and Wyllie, A. (1997). Becoming a Mother-An Analysis of Women's Experience of Early Motherhood. *Journal of Advanced Nursing, 25*(4), 719–728.

Barnes, M., Courtney, M., Pratt, J., and Walsh, A. (2004). The roles, responsibilities and professional development needs of child health nurses. *Focus on Health Professional Education: A Multi-disciplinary Journal, 6*(1) 52–63.

Barnes, M., Courtney, M., Pratt, J., and Walsh, A. (2003). Contemporary child health nursing practice: services provided and challenges faced in metropolitan and outer Brisbane areas. *Collegian, 10*(4), 14–19.

Bowden, P. (1997). *Caring. A gender-sensitive ethics.* London: Routledge.

Brooks-Gunn, J., and Chase-Lansdale, P. (1991). Children having children:Effects on the family system. *Pediatric Annals, 20*, 467–481.

Cronin, C., Shapiro, C., Casiro, O. and Chiang, M. (1995). The impact of very low-birth-weight infants on the family is long lasting: A matched control study. *Archives of Pediatrics and Adolescent Medicine, 149*: 151–158.

Deater-Deckard, K. (2004). *Parenting stress.* New Haven: Yale University Press.

Doucette, J. and Pinelli, J. (2004). The effects of family resources, coping, and strains on family adjustment 18 to 24 months after the NICU experience. *Advances in Neonatal Care, 4*(2): 92–104.

Dowd, N. (2000). *Redefining fatherhood.* New York: New York University Press.

Draper, J. (2003). Men's passage to fatherhood: an analysis of the contemporary relevance of transition theory. *Nursing Inquiry, 10*(1), 66–78.

Fägerskiöld, A. and Ek A-C. (2003). Expectations of the child health nurse in Sweden: two perspectives. *International Nursing Review, 50*, 119–128.

Feldman-Reichman, S., Millerm, A., Gordon, R. and Hendricks-Munoz, K M. (2000). Stress appraisal and coping in mothers of NICU infants. *Children's Health Care, 29*: 279–293.

Hays, S. (1996). *The cultural contradictions of motherhood.* New Haven: Yale University Press.

Heath, H. (2004). Assessing and delivering parent support. In M. Hoghughi, and N. Long (eds), *Handbook of parenting. Theory and research for practice* (pp. 311–333). London: Sage.

Higgins, I. and Dullow, A. (2003). Parental perceptions of having a baby in a neonatal intensive care unit. *Neonatal, Paediatric and Child Health Nursing* 6:3, 15–20.

Holditch-Davis, D. and Miles, M.S. (1997). Parenting the prematurely born child. *Annual Review of Nursing Research, 15*, 153–184.

House, J. (1981). *Work stress and social support.* Reading, MA: Addison-Wesley.

Jackson, K., Ternestedt, B.M. and Scholin, J. (2003). From alienation to familiarity: experiences of mothers and fathers of preterm infants. *Journal of Advanced Nursing, 4*(2), 120–129.

Kaila-Behm, A. and Vehviläinen-Julkunen, K. (2000). Ways of being a father: how first-time fathers and public health nurses perceive men as fathers. *International Journal of Nursing Studies*, 37, 199–205.

Marsiglio, W., Amato, P., Day, R. and Lamb, M. (2000). Scholarship on fatherhood in the 1990's and beyond. *Journal of Marriage and the Family, 62*, 1173–1191.

McCubbin, H. and Patterson, J. (1985). Adolescent stress, coping and adaptation: a normative family perspective. In G. Leigh, and G.W. Peterson (eds), *Adolescents in families* (pp. 256–276). Cincinnati, OH: Southwestern.

McKenry, P. and Price, S. (2000). Families coping with problems and change. In P. McKenry, and S. Price (eds), *Families and Change. Coping with stressful events and transitions* (pp. 1–21). Thousand Oaks, Cal.: Sage.

McVeigh, C and Smith, M. (2000). A comparison of adult and teenage mother's self esteem and satisfaction with social support. *Midwifery, 16*(4):269–276.

Miles, M.S., Funk, S. and Kasper, M. (1992). The stress response of mothers and fathers of preterm infants. *Research in Nursing and Health, 15*, 261–269.

Nolan, M. (1997). Antenatal education-where next? *Journal of Advanced Nursing, 25*(6):1198–1204.

Nyström, K. and Örhling, K. (2004). Parenthood experiences during the child's first year: literature review. *Journal of Advanced Nursing, 46*(3), 319–330.

Rice, P. L. and Naksook, C. (2001). Breast-feeding practices among Thai women in Australia. *Midwifery, 17*, 11–23.

Rane, T. and McBride, B. A. (2000). Identity theory as a guide to understanding father's involvement with their children. *Journal of Family Issues, 21*(3), 346–366.

Rogan, F., Schmied, V., Barclay, L., Everitt, L. and Wylie, A. (1997). 'Becoming a mother' – developing a new theory of early motherhood. *Journal of Advanced Nursing, 25*(5), 877–885.

Rowe, J. Gardner, G., and Gardner, A. (2005). Parenting a preterm infant: experiences in a regional neonatal health services program. *Neonatal Paediatric and Child Health Nursing, 8*(1), 17–23.

Rowe, J. and Barnes, M. (2006). The role of child health nurses in enhancing mothering know-how. *Collegian* 13(4).

Rowe, J. (2003). A room of their own: the social landscape of infant sleep. *Nursing Inquiry, 10*(3), 184–192.

Saggers, S. and Sims, M. (2005). Diversity: beyond the nuclear family. In M. Poole (ed.), *Family: Changing families, changing times* (pp. 66–87). Sydney: Allen and Unwin.

Singer, L., Salvator, A., Guo, S., Colin, M., Lilien, L. and Baley, J. (1999). Maternal psychological distress and parenting stress after the birth of a very low-birth-weight infant. *Journal of the American Medical Association, 281*(9): 799–805.

Singleton, A. (2005). Fathers: more than breadwinners? In M. Poole (ed.), *Families: Changing families, changing times.* Sydney: Allen and Unwin.

SmithBattle, L. (2003). Displacing the 'Rule Book' in caring for teen mothers. *Public Health Nursing, 20*(5), 369–376.

CHAPTER 5

Working It Out Together: Being Solution-Focused in the Way We Nurse with Children and Their Families

Bernie Carter

Overview

> Have you ever watched a beginner on the slabs? A most instructive little psychological study. He puts his foot on a hold which he doesn't like and then does his very best to prove to himself that he's right in not liking it. He fidgets about but he doesn't succeed in getting the foot to step off. So he develops a tremor and tries to shake it off. Still it stays firm so in desperation he gets on to it, lies flat against the rock and with a yell of triumph pushes. With the right direction of effort the mind of man can accomplish almost anything. (Perrin, 1985 citing Menlove Edwards, 1930)

There are probably very few chapters on children's nursing that start with a quotation from one of Britain's foremost climbers of the 1920s and 1930s. However, notwithstanding the rarity value of a climbing quotation in nursing books, it is a good place to start a chapter on Solution-Focused Nursing. Edwards was an extraordinary climber by the standards of his day, pushing the boundaries of what was thought to be possible and laying the foundations of modern climbing. He was imaginative, technically skilled and a great lateral thinker. When he looked at a crag – he saw possibilities, he saw ways up the rock-face and as he worked his way up the route he solved the challenges. What confounded him, as can be seen in his opening quote, is the way in which some novice climbers would approach 'the slabs' (a well-loved climbing area in North Wales) and problematize the route, convincing themselves that it was too hard, that the foothold too small. He notes that the act of believing that they couldn't do it, meant that they would eventually fall off (thus fulfilling their initial prophecy that they were right in thinking it was too hard).

So what's the connection between rock climbing and children's nursing? In particular, what has Menlove Edwards got to do with Solution-Focused Nursing? The simple answer to both these questions is 'Quite a lot.' Whilst most children's nurses (unless they are really lucky) won't be expected to climb high mountain crags, they are expected to provide nursing care for children and their families. The link is that children's nurses need to think more like Edwards and approach children/families with imagination, technical skill, enormous reserves of energy and lateral thinking. In other words we need to think in a more solution-focused way. The alternative is that we frame the children/families we work with as 'health problems.' The danger is that if all that we see are problems we are much more likely to fall off the (metaphorical) crag and we may also pull the children/families off with us.

Within this chapter, Solution-Focused Nursing (McAllister, 2003) is explored in the context of nursing children and their families. The case is made for the connection between Appreciative Inquiry (AI) and Solution Focused Children's Nursing (SFCN). AI is a framework for thinking appreciatively with people about situations and settings. It is well established as a way of bringing about organisational change and is becoming established as a way of guiding research. It also has many positive elements to offer nurses working with children and their families. These connections are explored and drawn out and contrasted with the more dominant problem oriented discourses.

Three stories are presented to help explore and extend understanding of the ways in which SFCN can extend and enhance children's nursing practice and the lives of children/families who are receiving nursing care. These stories provide opportunities for reflexivity, discussion and considering best practice.

Introduction

> To raise new questions, new possibilities, to regard old problems from a new angle, requires creative imagination and marks real advance in science. (Einstein and Infeld, 1938)

The history of children's nursing is one of change, revolution and the adoption of new paradigms. Each new era has resulted in different ways of nursing children, different philosophies of care, different technologies supporting care, different perceptions of the best setting in which children should be nursed, different approaches to and understandings of children and their families (see Davies, 2000; Alsop-Shields and Mohay, 2001).

Key changes have included moves from primarily hospital-based care to community based care; from an era when parents were banned from visiting to parent-led care; from a biomedical model to a holistic child (and family) centred model; from a hierarchical model to a model based on partnership, involvement and collaboration. Our view of children, reflecting that of society, has shifted from children being perceived as passive recipients of our expert care to much more as fellow citizens (de Winter *et al.*, 1999; Carter, 2002).

Yet within all these changes one key element has remained, until relatively recently, pretty much undisturbed; invisible and therefore forgotten or ignored. Children's nursing continues to adopt a more-or-less problem oriented approach to care. Whilst a problem-orientation is not wrong per se; it is, at its best, somewhat limiting. It can constrain our thinking and our practice. Being totally focused on the children's problems, even if we are judicious in the way in which we articulate these problems, is at odds with an holistic, partnership approach to caring for and, more importantly, caring with children and their families. We are in danger of seeing the problem and not the child.

Reader Activity: Locate (and enjoy reading) a copy of any one of the 'Joey Pizga' books by Jack Gantos. One of my favourites is 'Joey Pizga Swallowed the Key'.
Make notes as you go, about:

(a) who sees Joey as a problem and why they problematise him, and
(b) Joey's perspective on 'his problems' and the extent to which he agrees/disagrees with other people's opinions?

Now reflect on these two sets of notes and think about what you have learned about yourself, children like Joey and the way that adults sometimes view them.
What are the strengths and limitations of using a problem-oriented approach with Joey?
What are the effects on (a) him and his family, and (b) nurses and nursing?

As you will be able to see from working through the previous activity, there is a real dissonance between Joey who is a 'good kid' and other people's perceptions of him as a 'problem'. The same dissonance exists for children's nurses who claim to be working holistically and in partnership with parents/ children if their focus is on problems. The assumption within this approach, even if this is not conscious, expressed or explicit, is that nurses somehow know best or better than the child/family. We do not. Whilst we might know the disease and have insight into symptoms, symptom management and the psycho-social sequelae only the child and family know 'their illness'.

From Problem-busting to Sharing in Seeking Solutions

The shift from care acuity to care chronicity has heightened the imperative to move from being problem-oriented to solution-oriented. When genuinely supporting children with chronic ill health, children's nurses need to embrace and fully engage with the child's/family's specific expertise. Their expertise is based on their unique knowledge of living with, responding to and managing the multiple complexities of the everyday life-practices created by chronic illness (see Pelchat and Lefebvre, 2004 for a really good example of holistic, collaborative, transformative care). Children's nurses who move away from being primarily problem-busters can develop more creative, innovative practices as solution-supporters who help children and their families to 'live well' even if the child is sick. The notion of 'living well' is a relatively new concept that has emerged as societal attitudes and the dominant discourses about chronic illness have shifted.

I'm sure that Einstein did not have SFCN in mind when he talked about real advances being predicated on the ability to 'raise new questions, new possibilities' and use 'creative imagination.' However, these are the fundamental ingredients needed for children's nurses to ensure that acutely sick children and chronically ill children are not framed as problems needing nursing interventions. However, being solution focused is not just a simple shift; it requires a commitment. It requires practitioners to change their angle of perspective so that they don't automatically frame the world in terms of health care problems. This shift in perspective does not mean that the problems cease to exist – this is naive – but, (and this is a very big but), by focusing on solutions means they can be tackled in a very different way.

Adopting an affirmative, solution-oriented approach can be incredibly rewarding both personally and professionally. Taking an affirmative stance means that the mindsets of the nurse and child/family are firmly focused on what the child/family want to happen in the future, on what is already working well, on what they are doing to get their visioned future and how they know they are making progress (see Bowles *et al.*, 2001). Being solution-oriented is not an easy option; it requires us to develop a repertoire of sophisticated skills. Pirsig (1974) suggests that solutions are always simple once you've worked out what they are.

In the following story extracts it is possible to see the advantages of a solution-focused approach to nursing children and their families. The first two stories form part of a series of research interviews I undertook with parents in studies trying to understand parents' perspectives, experiences and expectations of health care professionals (Carter *et al.*, 2002). Story three, comes from a research study I undertook with children with complex health needs and with their siblings (Carter, in press).

The way I work as a narrative researcher draws on many of the same fundamental principles as those found in Solution-Focused Nursing. As a children's nurse researcher I know that the parents know far more than me about caring for their children at home and that despite my potentially greater academic, conceptual and theoretical knowledge, their experiential knowledge surpasses anything I possess. I strive to research with parents and the more time I spend with parents the greater respect I have for the skilled, nuanced care they provide their child on an ongoing/continuous basis. In particular I respect the way they can subtly shift their care in response to changes in the child's responsiveness, and symptoms and signs that might be overlooked by even the most expert children's nurse.

Jenny and Toby's Story

Toby is Jenny's first child. He was born prematurely, had a stormy first few weeks of life and was in a special care baby unit for several months before being discharged home. He continues to experience respiratory difficulties and chest infections.

> At the beginning, when I brought him home, there was no-one around really. He was tiny – just a little scrap and I was so ... frightened ... Toby had loads of chest infections that first year – I was desperate at times, really, really desperate for help. And then we got someone – a nurse. She had a lot of ideas and although I was grateful for there being someone at hand, she kind of took over a bit. I was kind of resentful .... I had been managing on my own quite well ... She did this assessment on me and Toby and then said she'd get some respite for me ... but I didn't really know what it would mean. I do get very tired with Toby with his feeds and things, but I don't want strangers looking after him ... he'd hate that .... But we got some respite and then the other service started and then I got some nursery hours. So it was like from nothing to loads of services, loads of people ... it was overwhelming. I wondered if I'd done something wrong to begin with – if she thought I couldn't cope with Toby ... I'd had no help for so long that I suddenly felt that I was drowning in a tidal wave of people and Toby got quite upset. They were all nice, they were good people but I didn't seem to have any control at all.

Reader Activity: Where did the nurse miss opportunities to use a solution focused approach to nursing? How did this make Jenny feel?

If you were now in the position of being Jenny and Toby's solution focused nurse, what would you do on your first few visits? Why? What would you be trying to achieve?

Critically reflect on your own practice. Do you ever start to take things over when it is not really appropriate? Make a note of when this happens (and why) and also make a note of what strategies you use to stop this happening (and whether or not they work).

Alice and Sam's Story

Alice is Sam's maternal grandmother and his primary care giver. She is married to Bryan and is talking about the support that she gets from Amy and Sarla (Sam's children's community nurses). Sam has a chronic and deteriorating neurological condition and his frequent seizures are not well controlled with medication. She describes how the nurses helped her manage Sam's gastrostomy tube and prepare her for Sam having a Mickey button inserted to help manage his feeds more easily.

> The nurses have been brilliant … his naso-gastric tube came out again, a week later. But he was brilliant. He let me put it in! … Amy and Sarla let me try and reassured me it wouldn't hurt Sam. They said if he got stressed or if I did didn't like it, I could stop and they'd give me a hand. And he sat there and Amy said 'Go on swallow'! And Sam did, you know. And it went straight down. They talked about things with me and Sam and it was so fine
>
> And Amy brought me all the things to show me about his gastrostomy and about having a Mickey button put in. And she said they could put the Mickey button in and measure him up … and they could show me … . But I just didn't feel that I could take that on – not at the moment anyway. So they've said, 'No worries, no hurry' – so I can get to that in a week or something – once I've thought about it – got my head round it and things … It's all a lot to take on you know.
>
> But yeah, they've been really good. Just there at the end of the phone. If you just want to talk and that. And they don't tell me what to do – not unless I really ask them that – they find out what I want and then we sort it out. Nothing's a trouble. They don't make me frightened – nothing like that – just calm and not winding the situation up. Sam's hard enough work as it is without everyone telling me 'Do this, do that'. … You can ask them anything, anything at all. They talk things through and I can tell them if I don't think something will work right with Sam. They are really experienced but Sam's a really special child – he needs things done a special way and I know what he needs.
>
> The main thing for me is knowing they're there. We haven't seen them for a couple of weeks – like the last time she said, 'there's nothing really for us to come to see you with' so she said, 'I'll leave it a little while, or we can come on a regular once a week basis if you like, but if you need us. …' She's left it all down to me and how confident I feel with what I'm doing but that's because they've showed me what to do.

Reader Activity: Identify what skills and knowledge Amy and Sarla are using in their interactions with Alice, Bryan and Sam. Are these skills that you have? Which of them would you like to develop most (and why)?

Why do you think Sam's family feels so positive about the children's nurses' involvement?

Amy and Sarla's seem to have prepared Sam effectively for replacement of his naso-gastric tube. Using a solution focused approach, how might you go about preparing Sam for his surgery and working with the family afterwards to continue to build their confidence and self-efficacy?

Subtle differences exist in the philosophical stance taken by each nurse in the two stories just discussed. Even though both stories reveal the intention by nurses to be helpful and resource-providing, in the first story, the mother felt overwhelmed and helpless, and in the second story, the mother felt empowered and capable. This difference illuminates a key point about being solution focused. Working 'with and for' clients, rather than 'on' them, requires a certain amount of power rebalancing. It's not about giving up one's expert knowledge, but it is about being conscious of the way expertise is transmitted. Expertise is not uni-directional, but a two-way possibility. In an SFN approach, effort is made to discover, work with and build up the person's capacities, to work with what's going right, and to help the person notice and value their strengths, so that they continue to feel optimistic and capable of enduring the difficult life circumstances.

Ella's Story

In the middle of visiting a family, Ella asked me a lot of questions about whether I had 'problems.' I was slightly fazed by these questions to begin with but I told Ella about my asthma and how it was bad sometimes but usually OK. A little while later Ella said in a very concerned voice:

> The nurses come to see Lily 'cos they say she's got problems ... problems with her tummy and her head and her feeding and fits and things. ... but she hasn't really got so many problems ... she's pretty special. She's not quite the same as us, but she's not much of a problem even though she does things different. She's my little sister

Reader Activity: How ethical is it to frame children as health care problems? What impacts might this have on the Lily's siblings and parents?

Clearly Lily does need support from nurses and health care professionals, what benefits for Lily and her family would accrue from working with Lily's family within a solution focused or appreciative framework?

What sort of story might you tell and share with Ella about 'special' children? How might you encourage Ella to tell her story?

So How Might We 'do' Solution-focused Children's Nursing?

Solution-Focused Nursing has similar values to Appreciative Inquiry (AI) (Watkins and Cooperrider, 2000; Van der Haar and Hosking, 2004). Although AI has primarily been used as an organizational change and/or research framework the fundamental principles that underly it are very consonant with nursing practice. It is as much a way of thinking as a way of doing. At its heart AI is an affirmative, dialogic, positive, relational way of developing best nursing practice with children and their families. It helps us contextualise illness within a family's lifeworld (see Hyde *et al.*, 2005).

As can be seen in the stories, there are major philosophical differences between a problem-oriented approach and a solution focused/appreciative approach. These philosophical differences are important since they result in very different ways of practising as a nurse and being-with families.

In Jenny and Toby's story, Jenny describes a 'good' nurse who identified a number of problems and sorted these out but who did not really make the situation any better. If anything Jenny feels worse about things even though she has more 'help'. In Alice and Sam's story, the initial situation is similar but the nurses' work in a much more solution-oriented way and they enable Alice to make decisions, to be in control and to identify their priorities. Alice becomes more confident and more resilient as a result of the nurses' involvement. Whilst they may 'do' less nursing in the traditional sense of the word, they are genuinely delivering high level, expert nursing care. In Ella's story the problem with problems is deftly explored by an eleven year old who has grasped the moral ambiguity of problem-centred care.

SFCN and appreciative nursing practice draws on what children and parents already do well with the aim of enhancing it and the skill set they already possess. Working within an AI framework means that practice (as well as research) can be seen as something to celebrate (Carter, 2006). Celebration is a compelling approach to practice. SFCN starts with accepting that if we explore with families their successes and achievements, potentials and capacities, competencies and energies, resources and assets, positive choices and strengths we are likely to discover what is already working and be able to move forward and

Table 5.1 Assumptions underpinning Appreciative Inquiry (AI) (Hammond, 1998) and Solution Focused Children's Nursing (SFCN)

AI is based on assumptions that:	*SFCN is based on assumptions that:*
In every society, organization or group, something works	In every family parents know what works best for them
What we focus on becomes our reality	What children and families focus on becomes their lived experience/reality
Reality is created in the moment, and there are multiple realities	The lived experience of being ill/sick or caring for a child who is sick is created in each moment of care or living; there are ways of experiencing things and multiple ways in which nurses can care with families.

Continued

Table 5.1 Continued

AI is based on assumptions that:	*SFCN is based on assumptions that:*
The art of asking questions of an organization or group influences the group in some way	The way in which nurses frame questions and the nature of those questions will affect the way the child and their family will view themselves and the nurse
People have more confidence and comfort to journey to the future (the unknown) when they carry forward parts of the past (the known)	Children and families can face a future in which their child is ill if they can draw on their past experiences and see that they have strengths and have capacity. Children's nurses can facilitate this
If we carry parts of the past forward, they should be what is best about the past	Nurses need to help families focus on the 'best of what has been' and to bring that with them, this will include their strengths, memories and their skills
It is important to value differences	It is important for children's nurses to value and respect diversity and individuality within and between families
The language we use creates our reality	The language children's nurses use can frame the way they and the families they 'care with' think, their expectations and their experiences. Framing language within a solution oriented paradigm is likely to create a more affirmative, dialogic, creative and aspirational approach to daily life practices

sustain their success(es). Hammond (1998) proposes a number of assumptions about AI and these can be transferred across and adopted by children's nursing (see Table 5.1).

Researchers working with AI draw on the 4-D cycle and this cycle could be transferred to SFCN to provide guidance for working with children and their families (see Table 5.2). The cycle consists of four phases – discovery (the best of what is or has been), dreaming (what might be), designing (what should be) and destiny (what will be) (Carter, 2006). The cycle starts with the choice of where to begin; this affirmative choice needs to be negotiated between the child/family and the nurse. It is important to remember that what we as nurses might see as a priority may not be the most important thing that the child/family wants to find a solution for.

Table 5.2 Using the AI 4-D cycle to guide Solution Focused Children's Nursing (SFCN) (developed from Carter, in press)

Discovery Phase	In this phase the nurse uses generative questions to trigger story telling about past experiences, memories and values. This needs the nurse to use careful listening and prompting skills. Amongst other things, the nurse needs to inquire, explore and appreciate: what makes things work well for children and their families what helps them feel positive, happy, motivated what they already know about getting things right This phase often includes the 'miracle question' in which the child/family are asked to imagine what things would be like if a miracle happened and the best was always happening. Using these stories explores the child/family's experiences and helps make sense of them and builds a comprehensive view of each child's/family's world as they understand and experience it.
Dream Phase	In this phase the nurse aims to explore with the child/family 'what might be' and to develop a strategic focus. In this phase 'the interview stories and insights get put to constructive use' (Cooperrider and Whitney, 1999). The nurse works with the child/family to come up with: a vision of how things could be better in the future. This is encapsulated in 'provocative propositions' (statements that realistically sum up 'what could be') created by the child/family/nurse. a powerful reason for achieving that vision a strategic statement that identifies how this migh be achieved
Design Phase	In the design phase the nurse and child/family focus on creating an ideal way of living with and managing the child's illness. This needs to be done within the context of their own family. This is based on grounded examples that have emerged from the successes and achievements that the family have had in the past.
Destiny Phase	In this phase a solution focused approach has become embedded and the child/family and nurse relate effectively with each other and they genuinely appreciate each other's strengths and capacities. This phase is focused on creating the networks and structures that facilitate connections and the potential to co-create new ways of 'living well' with the child's illness.

So What Does Solution-Focused Nursing Really Offer?

> And now here is my secret, a very simple secret: It is only with the heart that one can see rightly; what is essential is invisible to the eye'. (Antoine de Saint-Exupéry, 1985, *The little prince*)

Increasingly, children's nurses need to adopt a role in which they coach, guide, mentor, inform, share and work with children/families to develop the child's/family's skills, confidence, expertise, and knowledge (see for example, Carey, 2002; Hopia *et al.*, 2005). Children's nurses need to draw on all of their skills and judgement to devise, in collaboration with each child and their family the best individualized care possible; individualized in terms of it fitting in with and supporting the child's own specific health 'needs' as well as the child's/family's own life practices. Solution-Focused Nursing offers a philosophical framework, albeit one which is still emerging, which can provide direction and support to nurses who want to nurse differently, innovatively and with children/families.

Being focused on solutions rather than problems creates a climate in which we can engage with children's stories and generate closeness because we are in dialogue with them (Carter, 2004). It offers a move away from professional monologues, where we (nurses) – the so-called experts – 'colonize the lifeworld' (Porter, 1998) of children and parents who passively accept unidirectional interaction; where we talk to them and where they talk to us but where the meaning and the sense of what is said is not shared, explored and understood. We can co-construct meaning with families (Meiers and Tomlinson, 2003).

It offers an approach that allows us to be humble and aware that, despite our professional knowledge and expertise, we know very little in comparison to children's/parents' experiences of being ill and living with illness. As Bochner (2001, p. 149) states, storytelling makes an ethical claim on us 'for a dialogic relationship with a reader or listener that requires engagement from within, not analysis from outside, the story' (emphasis added). Many children want a dialogical relationship with health-care professionals. Their stories illustrate their desire to be involved, to understand more about their illness, their treatment and what is happening to them. By being reflexive and dialogic practitioners we can enter into children's 'cultures of communication' (Christensen, 2004).

Conclusion

As with any change in thinking, SFCN offers us a new way of framing and thinking about our practice as children's nurses (regardless of whether our role is clinical, managerial, academic or research). SFCN is not fully evolved; it's still at odds in many ways with the dominant (problem-oriented/needs-based) paradigm. However, just as with other revolutionary thinking the newly emerging ideas need forging and refining, thinking through and challenging, embracing and rejecting, and comparing and contrasting with the frame of reference we currently accept as the norm. What SFCN does offer is a new frame of reference whilst accepting that a problem-oriented approach continues to have value. It offers children's nurses a velvet gloved revolution; it does not smash problem based approaches but it offers an alternative. Being solution-focused, to a greater or lesser extent means thinking outside of conventional (often bio-medically oriented) approaches.

For many experienced and expert children's nurses solution-focused approaches will strike a chord with the way that they already practice since they will often have moved away from a binary thinking approach to a more creative, imaginative, boundary testing and pluralist way of working with children and families. For those children's nurses who are just starting our in their training, it offers a positive way of acknowledging the expertise, skills sets and competence of children and families. It offers a co-operative way of caring. It provides us with a more generous way of being children's nurses; a more generous – see Frank (2004) – (and reciprocally rewarding) way of caring. It opens up the possibilities that care is extended, ongoing, embracing and encompassing rather than packaged, measured, predictable and allocated. Because we, as children's nurses learn from the children and families we care for, we are able to develop more creative and imaginative ways of caring and creating solutions.

Group Activity: Prior to working together in a small group each of you will need to have collected three stories from a child (or from different children). Remember you will need to ask the child's and their parents' permission for any stories they tell to be shared in class. (You may also need permission from the nurse manager). Ask the child to tell you:

A story about them being involved in their care and what this felt like

A story about when they didn't feel that they were involved in their care and what this felt like

A story about what they would wish for if they had a magic wand they could wave over their nurses that would make the nurses 'the best nurses in the world'.

Remember you will need to think of appropriate wording to use, to ensure that the children of different ages/cognitive abilities understand what is expected. Make an exact note of the wording you used and reflect on your choice of words.

Write these stories down as soon as you can and use as many of the children's words as you possibly can. If the child wants to write their story down that is also fine. Make notes on how the child told you the story – What you felt like when they were telling you the story. Make notes on anything else that you think was important about the stories.

Share the stories with the other members of your group and listen carefully to each other's stories. What are the common themes that emerge from the stories? What are the differences? How do you feel as a group now you have listened to a few

stories? As a group identify and list as many solution-focused learning points as you can from the stories. Now, as a group, decide which ones are the most important ones (rank the learning points 1st, 2nd, 3rd and so on). Discuss why you have ranked the most important learning point first. Are you sure that this would be the most important one for the children? If not why not?
Now each member of the group should pick a different learning point to take forward and put into practice. (e.g, this might be 'I will listen more to what children say'). At your next group meeting feedback how easy or difficult it was for you to implement your learning point. Why was this so? How did using this learning point help enhance your practice? What difference did it make for the children and families for whom you are caring? This group work could continue until there has been more sharing and implementing of learning points.

Suggestions for Further Reading

Carter, B. (2004). Pain narratives and narrative practitioners: A plea for working 'in relation' with children experiencing pain. *Journal of Nursing Management, 12*, 210–216.

Gantos, J. (2000). *Joey Pizga swallowed the key*. London: Corgi Yearling Books.

Hammond, S. (1998). *The thin book of appreciative inquiry* (2nd ed.). Plano, TX: Thin Book Publishing.

References

Alsop-Shields, L. and Mohay, H. (2001). John Bowlby and James Robertson: theorists, scientists and crusaders for improvements in the care of children in hospital. *Journal of Advanced Nursing, 35*(1), 50–58.

Bochner, A. (2001). Narrative's Virtues. *Qualitative Inquiry, 7*(2), 131–157.

Bowles, N., Mackintosh, C. and Torn, A. (2001). Nurses' communication skills: an evaluation of the impact of solution-focused communication training. *Journal of Advanced Nursing, 36*(3), 347–354.

Carter, B. (2002). Children's participation in health-care in the UK – gesture, rhetoric or real involvement? *Bioethics Forum, 18*(3/4), 29–35.

Carter, B., McArthur, E. and Cunliffe, M. (2002). Dealing with uncertainty: parental assessment of pain in their children with profound special needs. *Journal of Advanced Nursing, 38*(5), 449–457.

Carter, B. (2004). Pain narratives and narrative practitioners: a plea for working 'in relation' with children experiencing pain. *Journal of Nursing Management, 12*, 210–216.Carter, B. (2006). 'One expertise among many' working appreciatively to make miracles instead of finding problems: using Appreciative Inquiry as a way of reframing research. *Journal of Research in Nursing. 11*(1), 48–63.

Carter, B. (2006). 'They've got to be as good as mum and dad': children with complex health care needs and their siblings' perceptions of a Diana Community Nursing Service. *Clinical Effectiveness in Nursing.*

Carey, L., Nicholson, B. and Fox, R. (2002). Maternal factors related to parenting young children with congenital heart disease. *Journal of Pediatric Nursing, 17*(3), 174–183.

Christensen, P. (2004). Children's participation in ethnographic research: issues pf power and representation. *Children and Society, 18*(2), 165–176.

Cooperrider, D. L. and Whitney, D. (1999). Appreciative Inquiry: a positive revolution in change. In Holman, P., Devane, T. (eds), The change handbook: group methods for shaping the future, (pp. 245–261). San Francisco, CA: Berrett-Koehler Publishers, Inc.

Davies, R. (2000). A celebration of 100 years' achievement in child health. *British Journal of Nursing, 9*(7), 423–428.

de Saint-Exupéry, A. (1985). *The little prince.* London: Heinemann.

de Winter, M., Baerveldt, C. and Kooistra, J. (1999). Enabling children: participation as a new perspective on child-health promotion. *Child Care, Health and Development, 25*(1), 15–25.

Einstein, and Infeld, L. (1938) *The Evolution of Physics.* New York, Simon & Schuster

Frank, A.W. (2004). *The renewal of generosity: Illness, medicine and how to live life.* Chicago, IL: The University of Chicago Press.

Gantos, J. (2000). *Joey Pizga swallowed the key.* London: Corgi Yearling Books.

Hammond, S. (1998). *The thin book of appreciative inquiry.* (2nd ed.). Plano, TX: Thin Book Publishing.

Hopia, H., Tomlinson, P. S., Paavilainen, E. and Åstedt-Kurki, P. (2005). Child in hospital: family experiences and expectations of how nurses can promote family health. *Journal of Clinical Nursing, 14*, 212–222.

Liebling, A., Ellliott, C. and Arnold, H. (2001). Transforming the prison: romantic optimism or appreciative realism? *Criminal Justice, 1*(2), 161–180.

McAllister, M. (2003). Doing practice differently: Solution-Focused Nursing. *Journal of Advanced Nursing, 41*(6), 528–535.

Meiers, S. and Tomlinson, P. (2003). Family-nurse co-construction of meaning: a central phenomenon of family caring. *Scandinavian Journal of Caring Sciences, 17*, 193–201.

Pelchat, D. and Lefebvre, H. (2004). A holistic intervention programme for families with a child with a disability. *Journal of Advanced Nursing, 48*(2), 124–131.

Perrin, J. (1985). *'Menlove' The Life of John Menlove Edwards.* London: Gollancz.

Pirsig, R. (1974). *Zen and the Art of Motorcycle Maintenance.* London: Vintage.

Porter, S. (1998). *Social Theory and Nursing Practice.* Basingstoke: Macmillan.

Van der Harr, D. and Hosking, D.M. (2004). Evaluating appreciative inquiry; a relational constructionist perspective. *Human Relations, 57*(8), 1017–1036.

Watkins, J. and Cooperrider, D. (2000). Appreciative Inquiry: a transformative paradigm. *OD Practitioner, 32*(1), 6–12. Accessed on the internet 15 May, 2005 at www.odnetwork.org/odponline/vol32n1/transformative.html

Wright, M. and Baker, A. (2005). The effects of appreciative inquiry interviews on staff in the UK National Health Service. *International Journal of Health Care Quality Assurance, 18*(1), 41–61.

CHAPTER 6

Learning Disabilities and Solution-Focused Nursing

Mike Musker

Overview

People with learning disabilities have special needs and very often nurses are called to care for them and their family. As children, and throughout their lives, people with learning disabilities may require particular support to facilitate learning, development, social integration and adaptation. Clients can require assistance to moderate behaviours, develop social skills and identify and achieve work, leisure and life-style interests. Clinicians who work with clients who have learning disabilities need to be sensitive to the key principles of rights, independence, choice and inclusion. Mike Musker, the author of this chapter will draw from his extensive clinical experience working with forensic clients who have learning disabilities to explain the complex nature of learning disabilities, historical changes in care and ways nurses can work 'with and for' clients, rather than on them. Important concepts to be explored in this chapter will include: ways of being facilitative, supportive and solution oriented; the importance of communication; seeing people as individuals – who may be able as well as sometimes disabled, as independent as well as sometimes dependent. Finally the chapter will explore the importance of advocacy and moving beyond a paternal approach to care, to an approach that sees people as citizens who have the right to be informed, engaged participants.

Learning Disability and Nursing in the Margins

The term 'learning disability' captures a wide range of people and conditions and is often associated with the term 'impairment'. Words such as idiots, imbeciles, retards and cretins were actually once legitimate medical terms, but are now used as insults in everyday language.

The field of learning disability provides perhaps the clearest example of stigmatizing medical labels, where the emphasis has been placed on identifying the problem rather than honouring the person and their potential. On one level it is understandable that the medical profession, trained to diagnose deficits, has a tendency to focus on the negative side of a client's condition (Klotz, 2004). Yet the effect for carers is that they see a health care profession preoccupied with what their child cannot and will not be able to do. This can be disheartening and depressing for parents and carers (Larson, 1998).

As previous chapters have emphasized, language is a powerful force for shaping social values and practices. When negative labels are strongly attached to a client or group, the effect is stigma. Stigma can lead to alienation, stereotyping, victimization and disempowerment. Society, and particularly the able-bodied amongst us has tended to create and maintain social barriers for people with learning disability (Ramcharan and Grant, 2001). The current term for stigma attached to disability is 'disablism'. For change to take place, Cooley and Salvaggio (2002) suggest that we need to ditch the 'dis' in disability.

Within the last twenty years, the rise of the consumer and rights movements has seen some important positive change for people with disabilities. It would seem that the voices of families and consumers are finally being heard. International bodies like the World Health Organisation are changing its policies to influence such discourse on disability (Imrie, 2004). Solution focused nursing may also help to turn the negative tide by working with clients and parents on what it is that they actually want to do.

Disability Nursing

Nursing people with learning disability is a highly specialized area that requires experience and specialised training (Mitchell, 2004). As children, and throughout their lives, people with learning disabilities may require particular support to facilitate learning, development, social integration and adaptation. Clients can require assistance to moderate behaviours that might be seen as anti-social, develop social and daily living skills and identify and achieve work, leisure and life-style interests. Clinicians who work with clients who have learning disabilities need to be sensitive to the key principles of rights, independence, choice and inclusion (DOH, UK, 2001).

Whilst deinstitutionalization and expanded community care has seen many benefits for people with chronic illnesses and disabilities, there are also challenges. Where once care was provided by nurses and located in institutions, now care has shifted to families, particularly women. Caring for any dependent person is a burden, but caring for someone with a learning disability is doubly hard. Carers may frequently find their role continuing for 30–50 years – they may find themselves caring for their disabled child from birth through to old age (Vagg, 1998). Many of these children also experience psychiatric as well as learning disabilities (Maes, Broekman, Dosen, and Nauts 2003). The reported prevalence of dual diagnosis varies between 10 and 39 per cent but this is likely to be under-reported (Deb, Thompson and Bright, 2001).

The person with a disability and their carers are likely to experience lifelong difficulties accessing the services they will require as they develop and their needs change. The services that most families take for granted often pose a challenge – from simply finding clothes to fit, or locating a suitable school, attending regularly and negotiating transport are all difficulties. Unlike raising able-bodied, able-minded children, caring does not stop in the teenage years. For some young people with disabilities, leaving home and gaining independence may not happen but a positive future is still possible. A study by Smythe and McConkey (2003) showed that children with a severe learning disability who were about to leave school were more optimistic about their job prospects and ideas around independent living than were their parents. The challenge for clinicians is to help bridge the gap between parents' and child's hopes and expectations.

At the time of young adulthood, new issues such as sexuality, independence and parents' freedom begin to emerge. Questions and fears for the future arise such as, what will happen when parents are no longer able to care for their children? How will the learning disabled person cope with the death of their parents? Who will go on caring for them?

Parents who have a child with learning disabilities frequently experience a roller coaster ride of emotions from grief, through to hopefulness and acceptance. They expect when they approach professionals to be offered solutions, support, and a positive attitude, yet are frequently met with the latest fad or trendy beliefs. For example, the parents of Elle, a young girl diagnosed with autism wrote:

> We expected to talk with wise and sympathetic people, wise because of a wide experience with sick children, sympathetic because it was their vocation to help those in trouble. We were amateurs. They were professionals. But we had, we thought, a common task. Unconsciously we expected to be welcomed, not as patients, but as collaborators in work of restoring this small flawed spirit. We were doing something terribly hard and we had been doing it quite alone. We wanted information and techniques. We wanted sympathy, not the soppy kind; we were grown up adults, but some evidence of fellow feeling, which ordinary doctors give readily enough. And, was it unreasonable – we wanted a little reassurance, a little recognition, a little praise. It never occurred to us that these expectations were naïve, that the gulf between parent and ministering institution must deliberately be kept unbridgeable ... . (Park 1982, pp. 142–143)

Some parents are even made to feel that what they have been doing for many years is wrong. Joan Vagg (1988, pp. 276–285) an author and a parent of two daughters with learning disabilities asks of us:

> Tread carefully and with sensitivity, assume nothing, approach each situation with an open mind uncluttered by pre-conceived, ill informed ideas, show interest without being patronizing, offer a listening ear without feeling under pressure to offer advice, show support without being judgemental, be realistic about the application of modern theories and parents' response to them, help where help is possible, and stop short of making empty promises.

In sum, many families struggle to find the support they need. Some local governments are responding to this need by employing unqualified staff such as care assistants or care agencies and thus nursing skills are being diluted and in some cases, even lost. For some family carers, the only valuable supports they receive are from other relatives or other parents in a similar position.

Being mindful of these common issues may help nurses become more aware of the impact that everyday interactions have with clients. A small act of kindness and a positive attitude can inspire, rather than disillusion people.

Listening to the needs and requirements of parents and clients is an important first step. Just as many moving 'testaments of life' have been able to influence policy makers and move them to care. Similarly, the story retold here aims to sensitise students of nursing to the importance of maintaining hope, and using creativity and reason to achieve positive outcomes for clients.

John's Story

This story is an example of how it is sometimes necessary to step away from the current chaos that comes from reacting to challenging behaviours, and using problem focussed thinking to begin to see the human being behind the problems. As this story shows, Institutions can sometimes create more problems than they solve.

A few years ago, I started work within a clinical team who worked with a group of patients considered, quite frankly, to be at the end of the line. This unit was located in the most secure institution in the United Kingdom. There was nowhere more secure for people diagnosed with learning disability and challenging behaviours, and the care could not be passed on to someone else – this was the last resort.

John was a particular challenge for nurses in the unit. He has congenital achondroplasia (dwarfism) which is combined with other complications such as a malformed palate and teeth, causing speech difficulties. His low IQ of 60 and communication difficulties may have been related to his congenital condition and long term institutionalization. John had for many years got into the habit of hiding in his room. Any attempts to persuade him to engage with other people would usually result in him becoming violent. Other asocial behaviours were that John would eat with his hands, sleep on the floor, refuse to shower and stockpile his room with trash. The clinical picture was made more complex because if staff ever attempted to interfere with this way of living John would bite, pull their hair, or break into a frenzy of punching and hitting.

As the newest team member, I was shocked at the lifestyle John had learnt to maintain and was able to see the situation with fresh eyes and without the experience of having been assaulted by John. It seemed to me that John had learned that to get his own way, he should communicate his wishes through aggression and attacks. For him the only control he had in this maximum security institution was his room. As a consequence, there was a lot of fear around caring for John and staff had begun to despair in the same way that I suspected John felt about his situation. Other clients accepted the way John behaved, and did not approach him, appreciating the fact that he wanted to be on his own. John's mum was his only visitor and she would visit around once per year. The extent of the visit consisted of John refusing to see her, or accepting his gifts and then walking out without any communication.

But I also noticed some positive aspects. John had developed a good relationship with a couple of key staff and they could intervene with John in ways that other team members were not permitted. For example, they could go into his room and remove some of the rubbish. The difference with these clinicians was that John had come to know them over many years and trusted them. Yet even these clinicians were only permitted to go so far, and were not immune from attack, as was sometimes demonstrated. It was clear to me that John was quite capable of communicating with others, even though he was slightly embarrassed by his speech impediment.

I began to see that if we continued to focus on reacting to John's problem behaviours, the likelihood was that he would continue in this pattern of anti-social, friendless, predictable and soul-less lifestyle for many years to come. With persistence, I had managed to gradually build a rapport with John and I was able to speak to him by standing at his doorway, but without intruding on his sanctuary, his place of safety.

Thinking how to care differently required a conscious effort to critically reflect on our own responses and then to access expert advice, and use creative flexible thinking. We saw that we were preoccupied with behaviour management and minimising risks, rather than working on containing, raising awareness, building resilience or engaging with John (McAllister, 2003). Another new member to our team was an experienced learning disability nurse who had just completed a course in behavioural nurse therapy. The specialist training looked at analysing behaviours, motivators, and reinforcers. She helped the team to see that many of John's behaviours were essentially a result of institutionalization, disempowerment and a long period of us using a problem-focused approach. John had maintained this lifestyle for almost a decade and it was going to require a leap of faith to create change.

So, we met as a team and tried to consider John's needs from his point of view. We asked ourselves a series of questions: What was he realistically capable of doing? Was he capable of being rehabilitated into the community? How could we think about John's aggression towards others in a solution-oriented way?

Our team proceeded to develop what became known as the empowerment model (Musker and Byrne, 1997). This model recognizes that it is sometimes necessary to initially take control of challenging behaviours in order to empower the individual toward a positive self-supporting, autonomous lifestyle. We acknowledged that managing violence needs some form of control, but this must be set in an empowering framework and a health promoting philosophy. Instead of continuing to be reactive toward the violent episodes, we determined to take total control and introduce John to a lifestyle that matched his potential, developing and returning autonomy at the earliest opportunity. The end result was profound.

We set ourselves some positive solution focused goals, challenging current concepts and beliefs by asking ourselves the following question: If there was a miracle, what would be John's real potential? (Stevenson *et al.*, 2003). In addition to reducing violent incidents, we determined that John was capable of:

- Eating with others
- Sleeping on a bed
- Having a clean room – personal space
- Showering daily
- Spending time with others on the ward
- Developing meaningful relationships
- Going to the rehabilitation centre
- Going to the social events in the hospital
- Going out into the community
- Eventually returning to the community to live independently

Perhaps these are simple concepts to you and me, but in a problem saturated context, seemed to be an impossible dream.

Helping John required determination, coordination, belief, and the stamina to withstand the initial violence and resistance. Our behavioural nurse therapist was able to measure the changes and provide the theoretical background about shaping target behaviours using positive reinforcement for desired behaviours, and to expect that undesired behaviours would increase before they were extinguished. The therapist warned us what to expect, but asked us to keep our eye on the long-term goal of positive outcomes: Solution-focussed nursing.

We planned his care using McAllister and Walsh's (2003) Care Framework (see Figure 6.1). We explained to John what was going to happen and we wanted him to be part of the positive approach and we expressed our genuine belief in him and in his capabilities. Bearing in mind John's IQ was around 60, even he understood in his calmer moments that we wanted to help him. We initially had to restrain John out of his room and he fought with nursing staff with his usual biting, kicking and spitting. We set very short-term goals, like staying with others for 1 hour then he was able to return to the safety of his room, eventually this would extend to half days. We placed a bed in his room, which at first he broke, but we replaced it with an unrippable thick mattress version that was made especially for him. We had to restrain him in the shower room and encouraged him to shower, which took a number of hours of persuasion, tact and experience. We had to use this strategy many times until John eventually would spontaneously shower once guided to the area. John was also asked to eat in the dining room and was encouraged to eat using a spoon initially. All of the appropriate behaviours above were gradually introduced and John began to enjoy the positive feedback from nursing staff. He started to develop relationships with lots of new staff and other patients whereas before he would retreat into his room. It got to the point whereby the majority of the time John was self-directing his own socialization and started to feel part of the ward community.

The team was amazed at his progress and we began to believe that our ultimate goal for John was indeed achievable – returning John to the community. But one day something terrible happened.

Out of the blue, John attacked a female member of staff by pulling her long hair and punching her in the face in a frenzied attack. Our hearts sunk. We began to doubt our solution-focused approach. We feared that we had put others at risk. Perhaps John was beyond help. But once again the behavioural nurse therapist provided much needed motivation. She explained that that this behaviour was a common feature of creating change – there were bound to be a few spikes along the way. We reminded ourselves that John had lived this way for many years, and that we should expect our miracle to take a little more time.

Without reverting to old response patterns of containing the violence, we determined to assist John to reflect on what had led to the incident, the effect that his behaviour had had on the nurse and to remain positive about his recent progress. He was remorseful for his violent outburst wanting to retreat into his shell and wanting to apologize to the nurse he had assaulted. We assisted him to work through this episode, and just as the therapist had promised, violence became a rare event.

Eventually, after attending occupational therapy workshops, social events, and developing meaningful relationships with others, we were able to take John for days out into the community. A key marker for our team was the day John's mother was able to visit him, and she could not believe the difference in him. Being able to sit in a room on her own with her son was a major milestone. John developed a particularly strong relationship with one nurse and would go to great lengths to impress him. Days out became the ultimate reward for him and once these started we saw no more violent behaviour.

The remarkable transformation culminated in being able to discharge John to the community where he maintains his own apartment and receives ongoing support from a Management Assessment Panel (Mansell and Beadle-Brown, 2004). This panel meets to create community based plans for clients identified to have exceptional needs. John continues to do well.

Putting Principles into Practice

Essentially John's story was about doing leadership and doing nursing differently. As Thyer (2003) explained, transformational leadership involves being visionary, creative and providing positive reinforcement. The team that worked so well with John was multi-disciplinary. We learned that other professions respect nurses as equal and as such we are well placed to role model for them new ways of communicating and thinking, moving away from the plateau of problem centeredness that flourishes in medically oriented institutions (Bowles *et al.*, 2001).

Lipkin (2003) offers some other inspirational ways to create positive attitudes with people you work with and care for. These strategies may be useful to refocus and reframe the thinking of your team.

1. Stay brutally optimistic – see opportunities rather than difficulties. If you can see a solution, stand up and be heard.
2. Identify the most powerful benefit you offer to people around you and deliver it – make a meaningful contribution that you are proud of and learn to excite others with your ideas.
3. Pump up your personal vitality – be an energy source for other people, be visionary and inspire.
4. Be habitually generous – don't just consider reciprocity, exceed the expectations of others and lead the way.
5. Take control of your destiny – be the nurse you want to be, don't be submissive to cultures and professional boundaries. Value your ideas (adapted from Lipkin, 2003).

Applying the CARE model

The solution-focused interventions used in John's story can be summarised and explained using the CARE model described by McAllister and Walsh (2003).

We attempted to provide containment. Providing a safe secure environment for John was our initial aim, which meant initially providing some controls in the environment. The controls, however, were set in a clear positive path toward empowering John and staff had been provided with training about

C Containment- through accurate, helpful diagnosis, provision of safety, relief of symptoms and promotion of inner security.

A Awareness- aiming for self-awareness and insight through learning, self-reflection, safe recall, expression, storing memories, understanding and acceptance.

R Resilience- refocusing on personal strengths and abilities necessary for a full, meaningful, connected and peaceful future and recruiting self and others to build and sustain changes for a more integrated and accepting community.

E Engagement- building a trusting partnership through listening, empathising conveying hope and concern, motivating the person to do the work necessary to achieve self-understanding and facilitating a sense of meaning and manageability in the illness or recovery experience.

Figure 6.1 The CARE framework (McAllister and Walsh, 2003)

values led practice and empowering consumers. It is recommended that training be provided to mental health nurses to develop active therapeutic engagement and to develop a therapeutic milieu that is based on an evidenced based model (Stevenson *et al.*, 2003). All interventions that appeared coercive in nature were measured against behavioural improvements, although it was our gut instincts that led the way forward.

We also worked to raise awareness. For our team, awareness was a two-way street in that we had to acknowledge our own fears about being attacked, and John had to acknowledge what his desires were, and what he really wanted to be like in his ward community setting. We were able to tease out what John really liked and this included, some time to himself, going for walks in the grounds, going to the shop to buy sweets, and even helping staff with chores. This was achieved through a structured behavioural analysis through interview and observation. The key factor that was noted from the beginning was how shy John had become; it was similar to the feeling expressed in agoraphobia. It was necessary to invest in the belief that at the core nature of human beings, they are well intentioned.

We worked to build John's resilience. We were confident that John had the potential to live successfully in his ward community with others. He had learnt a pattern of behaviour that had become entrenched, so we understood the need to move gradually toward independent living. Even the longest journeys start with the first step. Over the six month period, balanced steps were being taken, and each time it was evident that John's resilience was increasing. A daily chart was completed which recorded both adaptive and maladaptive behaviours. Time sampling of behaviours, which involves more in-depth recording, showed marked improvements. It became evident that John had started to initiate conversations and was enjoying the experience of being with other people.

Throughout our approach to working with John, we focused on engagement. John developed a special relationship with two nurses and these became the anchors for positive change. He was eager to please them by demonstrating his progress, eager to show them he had cleaned his room, or to explain to them that he had had his shower. These special relationships were nurtured and became reciprocal in that the nurses would take John out for day trips, and spend extra time with him. It became necessary to make sure that part of the rehabilitation programme required investment in disengagement of the relationships that had been developed. Part of this process included visiting John in his new home, and allowing him to make calls back to the ward, ensuring a smooth transition.

Returning to the Community

Community resources for people with learning disability are few; sometimes every resource has to be fought for. One solution is to bring multidisciplinary agencies together and to encourage them to agree to share resources in a way that will benefit all stakeholders: A system known as Person Centred-Action

Planning (Mansell and Beadle-Brown, 2004). Some local governments (e.g. South Australia) have developed a Management Assessment Panel, which meets to create community based plans for clients identified to have exceptional needs. This is a government agency that helps people with complex community access issues, such as finding supported housing accommodation and supportive care in their home. The panel requests the attendance of stakeholders who can influence access to community resources and people who are currently involved in the patient's care. These include a variety of government, non-government agencies, the client and family. The panel facilitates a meeting, which includes the development of a resource plan, identifying future support to be provided by each agency. An example would include the allocation of a certain amount of 'face to face' hours in the client's home, or agreement on what access to day centres is available in their area. Stakeholders are asked to agree on their level of support and participation toward the development of a successful action plan. Another initiative to supporting a person's transition into the community is the use of a re-settlement facilitator. A person specifically employed to work between agencies, encouraging inter-sectoral and inter-organisational collaboration.

Group Activity: Values Led Practice: Make a list of all the things you have enjoyed doing over the last week/month and list them on a whiteboard as a group.
Identify whether the people you care for have access to the same facilities you have listed, like cinemas, hairdressers, mobile phones, and other activities that you have listed.
If not, how can you positively change practice to ensure access to such community facilities?

Suggestions for Further Reading

Larson, E. (1998). Reframing the meaning of disability to families: The embrace of paradox. *Social Science Medicine, 47*(7), 865–875.

Musker, M. (2001). Learning disability. Chapter 15 in, C. Dale, T. Thompson and P. Woods. *Forensic Mental Health, Issues in Practice* (pp. 161–168). Edinburgh: Bailliere Tindall.

Teacher notes to accompany this chapter can be found at www.palgrave.com/ nursinghealth/mcallister

References

Bowles, N., Mackintosh, C. and Torn, A. (2001). Nurses' communication skills: an evaluation of the impact of solution-focussed communication training. *Journal of Advanced Nursing, 36*(3), 347–354.

Cooley, B. and Salvaggio, R. (2002). Ditching the 'dis' in disability: supervising students who have a disability. *Australian Social Work, 55*(1), 50–59.

Deb, S., Thomas, M. and Bright, C. (2001). Mental disorder in adults with intellectual disability. 1: Prevalence of functional psychiatric illness among a community-based population aged between 16 and 64 years.*Journal of Intellectual Disability Research, 45*(6), 495–505.

Hassiotis, A. (2004). Developmental psychiatry and intellectual disabilities: An American Perspective. *British Journal of Learning Disabilities, 32*, 39–42.

Imrie, R. (2004). Demystifying disability: a review of the international classification of functioning, disability and health. *Sociology of Health & Illness, 26*(3), 287–305.

Jahoda, A. and Markova, I. (2004). Coping with social stigma: people with intellectual disabilities moving from institutions and family home. *Journal of Intellectual Disability Research, 48*(part 8), 719–729.

Klotz, J. (2004). Sociocultural study of intellectual disability: Moving beyond labelling and social constructionist perspectives. *British Journal of Learning Disabilities, 32*, 93–104.

Larson, E. (1998). Reframing the meaning of disability to families: The embrace of paradox. *Social Science Medicine, 47*(7), 865–875.

Lipkin, M. (2003). Ten researched ways to unleash the leader within you. *Canadian Manager, Spring*, 8–19.

Maes, B., Broekman, T., Dosen, A., and Nauts, J. (2003). Caregiving burden of families looking after persons with intellectual disability and behavioural or psychiatric problems. *Journal of Intellectual Disability Research, 47*(September, Part 6), 447–455.

Mansell, J. and Beadle-Brown, J. (2004). Person-centred planning or person centred action? Policy and practice in intellectual disability services. *Journal of Applied Research in Intellectual Disabilities,17*, 1–9.

McAllister, M. (2003). Doing practice differently: solution-focused nursing. *Journal of Advanced Nursing, 41*(6), 528–535.

McAllister, M. and Walsh, K. (2003). CARE: A framework for mental health practice. *Journal of Psychiatric and Mental health Nursing, 10*, 39–48.

Mitchell, D. (2004). Learning disability nursing. *British Journal of Learning Disabilities, 32*, 115–118.

Musker, M. and Byrne, M. (1997). Applying empowerment in mental health practice. *Nursing Standard, 11*(31), 45–47.

Park, C. (1982). *The siege.* Boston: Little, Brown and Company.

Ramcharan, P. and Grant, G. (2001). Views and experiences of people with intellectual disabilities and their families: the user perspective. *Journal of Applied Research in Intellectual Disabilities, 14*, 348–363.

Smythe, M. and McConkey, R. (2003). Future aspirations of students with severe learning disabilities and of their parents on leaving special schooling. *British Journal of Learning Disabilities, 31*, 54–59.

Stevenson, C., Jackson, S. and Barker, P. (2003). Finding solutions through empowerment: a preliminary study of a solution-orientated approach to nursing in acute psychiatric settings. *Journal of Psychiatric and Mental Health Nursing, 10*, 688–696.

Thyer, G. (2003). Dare to be different: transformational leadership may hold the key to reducing the nursing shortage. *Journal of Nursing Management, 11*, 73–79.

Vagg, J. (1998). Chapter 17, A lifetime of caring. In, T. Thompson and P. Mathias. *Standards and Learning Disability*, (pp. 276–285). London: Bailliere Tindall.

CHAPTER 7

Youth Work

Margaret McAllister

Overview

Many young people experience transitional crises when moving from youth to adulthood. The issues they face include forming identity, finding their own voice, finding places to belong socially and spiritually, tolerating confusion and flux, maintaining social connections and self-esteem, and developing a sense of meaning and manageability throughout dynamic and stressful periods of change. Some of the challenges for nurses working with youth include developing rapport and engagement, helping young people find their voice and use it effectively and assertively, supporting young people so that they feel able to bear emotional intensity and to see life's turning points as exciting rather than overwhelming.

For young people in distress or struggling to cope with social issues, solution focused approaches help to 'thicken up alternate stories' of being, so that they can see their lives filled with possibilities rather than obstacles (White and Epston, 1990). This chapter explores a story concerning self-harm, a common phenomenon amongst youth, to show how nurses working with young people are able to engage, listen, voice, validate and motivate for change.

Simon's Story

I remember sitting in the Activity room one morning waiting for handover. Simon, a 15 year old boy was sitting with me talking about the art work he had drawn the previous evening. I asked Simon if I could look at it, he agreed and walked to his room to retrieve it. Simon has a diagnosis of Adjustment Disorder, with depressed mood. A few days ago, he was admitted to our acute unit, via ambulance, for the management of a serious self-harm attempt. Over the past few months his teacher, Mrs Jones, had noticed that he had changed from being a happy, involved student, to one who was isolated and moody. He would ask her, 'What's the point of doing this assignment? What's the point of anything?'. Then one day, he looked agitated and asked if he could leave the room and sit outside. When the teacher went to attend to him, she found him curled up in a foetal position on the ground, blood seeping on to the pavement. Simon had used the point of a compass to lacerate both forearms. He was wailing, 'No one understands me, Mum doesn't love me, now Michael thinks I'm a freak. No one knows who I am!'

So this day, the picture that had attracted my attention was a charcoal drawing of a boy lying wide-eyed in a grave, complete with tombstone and inscription, 'Here Lies Sad Simon'. I asked Simon why he drew the picture and he replied, 'Because that's me, I feel like a dead person. I feel nothing any more'. At the time, I didn't say much more to Simon. I really didn't know how to respond.

But later, reflecting on the interaction and on the drawing, I tried to look beyond the surface level meaning of the grave, the inscription and the hint about suicide, to try to connect with the emotion. I could feel the boy's helplessness. But his eyes were open, and so I sensed that he didn't want to be dead, or in such a desperate, desolate position. To me Simon's drawing revealed a little spark of hopefulness. He was reaching out. I thought that his drawing could be a metaphor that together we could reframe.

The next time I met with Simon, I asked him if he wanted to know what I saw in his drawing, since the meaning of art is after all in the eye of the beholder. In this way, I had piqued his curiosity and he agreed to listen. I said that the image made me think about feeling frightened of being alone, being stuck in a dark place where there is no clear view, and feeling unable to get out of the situation without help. By now, he was nodding in agreement, and so I felt I could go on. I said I had a hunch, and would he mind me testing it out. Again he agreed and so I suggested, 'If you have bad feelings such as these expressed in your drawing, then maybe it's possible to have good feelings too?' He nodded, a little tentatively. I went on, 'Imagine, if you can, that boy in the picture being helped out of the pit, breathing easier, seeing things clearly, feeling safe. Imagine holding someone's hand, someone helping him out ... maybe, if you're interested, that's something you and I could work on doing together. Perhaps you could think about that for a while'... and that really was the beginning of how we started working together.

As it turned out, Simon worked through his feelings of being different, feeling like no one cared or understood, and he was able to see that he needed to take more time to understand himself and his changing feelings. After 10 days acute care, Simon was followed up in the community and during this time came to terms with a number of realizations – that he was gay, that he could help others, such as his mother and a good friend, understand his identity, rather than to try to tolerate their prejudice. He also learned that he could turn shame into pride.

Facilitating Healthy Transition in Adolescence

Adolescence, even for healthy happy, emotionally secure children, can be a time of multiple transitions and pose dilemmas for young people. There is the move from childhood to adulthood, from school to employment, from family social activities to peer group activities. It is a time of active exploration, of changeable behaviour, and of searching for meaning and place. No longer children, adolescents are in a transition space that is thinly described for them and about them. That is, public knowledge about what it means to be a child and what it means to be an adult are common sense and stable areas of knowing. But what it means to be an adolescent, remains ambiguous and poorly understood.

Indeed, many of the common experiences of youth are conveyed in ways that lead to a closing down of conversation with young people, so that many feel they have been wrongly judged or unfairly constrained. This is exactly what the generation gap is all about. In this gap, many adults fail to treat young people with respect, understanding or sometimes even basic humanity. Young people may be exploited, overlooked or dominated. Myths and stereotypes about young people abound.

Too often, young people complain that they have not been adequately heard, they have been patronized, or controlled by others. These were certainly feelings experienced by Simon. Within the story there is evidence of the nurse making a concerted attempt to open up conversation. The charcoal drawing became the conduit.

Reader Activity: Try to recollect a particular incident from your own teen age years and write an account of what you felt. Perhaps you could use these questions as a guide:

Do you recall what you thought about, how you felt?

Do you remember being aware of what it was like expressing different values and opinions to that of your family or school teachers?

Do you remember noticing that you were changing, and yet also feeling not sure of yourself and of your goals?

Because adolescence is a transition space between childhood and adulthood, the experience can be confusing, especially for the young person going through it. It is a time for emotions to be extreme or labile, for physical and social changes to be taking place that create uncertainty. And change isn't always a smooth process. Values, spirituality, morality and ethics are being put to the test for the young person whose world is opening up, and who may be being confronted with social groups and cultures that think and behave differently from what they have become used to. Adolescence can also be a time when the person suddenly takes hold of strong convictions and then perhaps just as easily lets them go. This changeability is often criticized and invalidated by a dominant group that unrealistically expects consistency. Rather, older adults, and young people themselves could be seeing this time of change as acceptable and for ambivalence to be expected.

Psychologists typically focus on the task of identity formation during adolescence, and this is not a simple undertaking for young people. Finding out the big life questions of 'who am I', 'what do I believe', 'what and how do I want to be', 'who do I want to be with' seem so much more complicated in the twenty-first century than they did in times when choices were more narrow and the global village was more a dream than a reality. It is useful to reflect on what has changed in the world, at least from the Australian point of view, over the last 40 to 50 years, so that one can more fully appreciate the unique challenges facing young people today.

The Contemporary World

This is now a conflict-ridden world. Violence and the threat of violence is everywhere, and at the forefront of most peoples' consciousness. We know through the media and every-day conversations that people are concerned about war, terrorism, violence in the movies, on television and in video games, domestic violence, date rape, bullying, road-rage and other crimes against people.

This is also a world in which information and access to knowledge has virtually exploded so that people can access huge amounts of information quickly and easily, relatively regardless of privilege, geography, gender, culture or class. The information-technology age has made the world a global village so that countries and cultures can be brought together. It offers the potential for many more people to access knowledge, and thus power. People have greater exposure to the richness and diversity of other cultures yet they are also confronted with more differences.

The civil rights and feminist movements have advanced awareness about the effects of oppression on marginalized groups, so that publicly at least, these differences are acknowledged and freedoms and opportunities have expanded for many social groups. Yet exploitation still occurs because dominant groups continue to be the ruling class, to enjoy the majority of the world's resources and to control the major socializing structures, such as schools and media that shape opinions and values. This issue is relevant to Simon's experience of perceiving difference and acknowledging his sexuality. Discussion of such social changes, the struggle and the various ways difference can be enriching can lead to discussion of strategies for empowerment in ways that are a little more distanced from personal experiences, and thus less confronting.

The quality of education provided to children and young people has also improved significantly. Educational discourse, both formal and informal, is flourishing and practical. It has clarified processes for achieving literacy and numeracy in most children, although children from indigenous cultures and low socio-economic groups remain disadvantaged. But it is timely to remember that it has only been in the last 40 years or so that High School has been an opportunity available for all young people, regardless of ability or finances. So, young people are on the whole, better educated, more literate, and potentially more discerning and reflective. Yet, they are faced with a much more sophisticated and seductive consumer world where advertising and subliminal messages compete with a person's capacity to be critical and questioning. The consumer society is successfully producing unquestioning acceptance of, and even attraction to, the superficial and the predictable. This is explained in the notion of the McDonaldization of society (Ritzer, 1993), in which, '... the process by which the principles of the fast-food restaurant are coming to dominate more and more sectors of American society as well as the rest of the world'. While this consumer society provides some conveniences such as variety, round-the-clock banking and shopping and often speedier service; there is a sense that this system is tending to turn in on itself, leading to irrational outcomes. Such outcomes are the replacement of human skills with non-human technology, the focus on quantity over quality, on efficiency over effectiveness, the worker who is not required to think and the dilution of ways people can be brought together through food preparation and eating rituals, through talking with service providers and not machines. This may be leading to a meaning-poor society and thus young people prepared with more education and more access to information, are challenged and stimulated less. Perhaps this in part explains the growing frustration, sense of being dissatisfied, experiences of depression and anxiety in young people.

While there is no evidence that Simon experienced this tension, it remains a useful issue to explore with him and other young people because it may further encourage him to remain conscious of the world around him and perhaps to see the value in mindfulness, rather than mindless conformity. Being critical, rather than passive to such social issues, may also be a way of promoting efficacy in young people, helping them to notice ways of using every-day activities such as being a discerning shopper to be political. In this way too, someone like Simon may be reminded that he does have power and that he can be influential.

At the same time as this meaning-poor culture is expanding, there is a loss of faith in organized religion and this has called some to question whether people really believe in anything of any depth anymore (Welton, 1995). It is also not a time of certainty or consistency. Full employment is now not a realistic platform for politicians to promise. People don't usually stay in one job for their whole career and nor will it mean that working can guarantee quality of life. And further, despite the amount of relatively cheap entertainment and variety of leisure activities available to people, more people are living isolated, disconnected and unhappy lives.

Ordinarily, one should expect that adolescence should be the healthiest time for a human being. In the early twentieth century, the major concern in relation to adolescent health was the treatment of infectious diseases, but now it relates to the effects of environmental and social factors (Bryan and Batch, 2002). According to a recent Australian national survey of mental health and well being, 13.4 per cent of boys aged 13–17 and 12.8 per cent of girls of the same age, experience mental health problems or disorders (Sawyer *et al.*, 2000).

Suicide and depression amongst young people are increasing. For those living in single-parent families and others in lower socio-economic circumstances, risks are even greater (Bryan and Batch, 2002). Drugs, such as alcohol, tobacco, marijuhana and amphetamines, are being used more frequently. Risk-taking behaviour, which offers the potential for enhanced feelings of self-esteem and peer respect, also carries the chance of negative effects. While on the one hand it is understandable that young people are likely to experiment with drugs, drug misuse can also signal psychological or social difficulties (Kang, 2002). Binge drinking is much more common in teenagers. In Australia from 1990–1997, more than half of all serious alcohol-related road injuries involved people aged 15–24 (National Drug Research Institute, 2001). About one quarter of deaths among Australians aged 12–24 were drug related (Kang, 2002). Sexual health issues such as unsafe sex, sexual assault and communicable diseases are also a concern.

So the world is complex and challenging and young people moving from childhood into this realm require at the very least skills in adjustment, because they are moving from the familiar to the new. Making a successful transition depends on whether the young person can find the changes and the challenges meaningful, manageable and worthwhile. Strong family, school and social supports, productive peer activities, a community that understands and expects changeability and flux and a young person armed with optimism, hope, resilience and inner strength are all needed. These are all protective factors identified as being effective in preventing the onset of illness and maintaining health and well-being (Rapp, 1989).

Reader Activity: While adolescence carries a lot of potential for tension, it is also a fabulous time for adventure and new experiences. Make a list of all the wonderful things you did as an adolescent. What effect did this have on your sense of self, your relationships with others and your future? Think about what this says about adolescence as a transition period.

Family

All people, if they are to thrive, need to feel safe, supervised and nurtured. Young people depend on a stable family environment in which there are sufficient boundaries and rules for the person to know limits and learn discipline. Parents in the family can do a great deal to moderate the effects of stress a young person may experience. They can be warm and supportive, communicative, responsive to the young person's needs, exert firm, consistent control and fair discipline and monitor the person's activities closely (Hetherington and Stanley-Hagan, 1999).

If problems are beginning to emerge, prevention and early intervention is available and it is effective. Parents can learn skills of effective parenting through such services as Triple P – the Positive Parenting Program, which effectively reduces risk factors associated with the development of various mental and social problems such as antisocial behaviour and youth suicide (Sanders *et al.*, 2003). Beginning in Queensland, this program is now available in the whole of Australia, New Zealand, Germany, the UK and the US. The program leads to children becoming polite, friendly and sociable, learning to control their emotions and developing problem solving skills. The program shows parents how to parent and also targets at risk groups.

What happens in the family is vital for social well-being. The quality of the family experience has a direct flow on effect to the wider community. Family conflict can leave adults and children feeling angry, depressed, unloved and powerless and those problems can be taken to work and school, where they continue to have a negative effect. We know that breakdowns in family relationships is linked to significant health and social problems. So the action taken here within this small social group has a lasting and significant effect on the health of our whole community. Working respectfully with family members is therefore clearly relevant to youth work.

School

Another protective factor is a positive school environment. Young people are still learning and developing and therefore depend on schools for socialization and healthy development. If those schools lack structured opportunities to learn, lack a sense that they value the input of the student, have bullying or unsafe conditions, then school fails to offer the protection and support young people need to grow and learn (Burns and Hickie, 2002).

In Australia, mental health promotion and illness prevention is now a national priority and many innovative school-based programs are developing. 'Mind Matters' (Dept of Health and Aged Care, 2000) provides hard copy information on issues to raise mental health literacy for secondary schools. 'Beyond Blue' (www.beyondblue.org.au) is an Australian website that offers a school based program designed to reduce depression, anxiety and substance abuse in young people and promote well being. There are also school based youth health nurses that can take an active role in establishing these school resources and in developing relationships with teachers and students. Whilst these resources were not available for Simon, they are something that could be put in place for the future.

Social Networks

Secure, supportive social networks are also crucial. Without them, the young person may be unable to form attachments and establish a feeling of connectedness. They may feel isolated, and lack opportunity to learn through role models and sharing of ideas. In Simon's case a critical moment in his life occurred when he became aware of feeling judged or misunderstood by his friend Michael and his mother and without their support, he had less capacity to cope. He experienced a crisis and his repertoire of productive coping strategies failed him. Social networks are needed to assist a young person to feel issues are manageable, depend on the support of others, sustain their identity, self-esteem and sense of stability.

Social attachment and connectedness are protective factors that are amenable to intervention. Nurses can work on enhancing the young person's skills in communicating and coping. Nurses can promote safe, secure environments, and find ways to value and validate a young person's contribution that they make to a community. Nurses need to be attuned to the power of friendships, to find ways to build up fragile and new identities, find ways for a young person to feel worthwhile, to understand difference in cultures, sub-cultures and generation gaps, and also engage with youth in their dilemmas, and work in partnership with them.

Community Partnerships

Community partnerships are also now recognized as an important health promotion strategy that can build understanding, keep young people connected to social supports and emphasize the value in maintaining and sustaining an environment conducive to well-being. When partnerships are in place, the level of supports involved with the well-being of young people is broadened. Partnerships also enable skills and resources to be pooled and are more powerful in advocating for positive change. Young people who have health or social needs can not be adequately helped in one service alone. It requires a whole of community response if we are serious about systematic change. And such change is possible, for as Margaret Mead (1901–1978) once poignantly said,

> Never doubt that a small group of thoughtful, committed citizens can change the world. Indeed, it is the only thing that ever has.

And with the renewed focus on community health promotion, one of the effective ways of encouraging citizens to change the world so that is more youth-friendly is to work on expanding mental health literacy (Meadows and Singh, 2001). This is one of the new buzzwords for working with communities.

Where 'being literate' means having the ability to fluently read a text, mental health literacy refers to understanding terms, treatments, needs and recovery strategies that prevent mental illness and enhance mental health. Becoming literate is important for communities, because it may help us all to be alert to practices that stigmatize or harm people by limiting their recovery and social integration. No longer are youth workers and mental health experts focused totally on an individual's treatment needs. Working with communities to develop their mental health literacy is now considered equally important. This work involves changing knowledge and attitudes to encourage better health service utilization and greater acceptance of young peoples' unique needs.

It is useful to imagine a community as young-people friendly and one that has strong literacy skills. This is a community that has knowledge and awareness of mental health symptoms and the factors that can reduce risk of ill-health. This is a community that values help-seeking behaviour in young people, and their family and friends, the skills of health professionals and effective treatments and self-help. This is a community that resources and develops services that provide education and support for affected people and a range of networks and services for young people including sport and recreation, entertainment and leisure skills, health and well-being, employment, accommodation, spiritual and meaning rich environments. School based youth health nurses and other youth workers can use this image of community to focus their work and provide rationale for why community education, and information campaigns can be important and effective parts of their role.

Cultivating Inner Strength and Spirit(uality)

There is much that we can do to develop environments that are spiritual and meaning rich. Webber (2002) provides some helpful insights about understanding the potential that spirituality has for giving hope to young people in the face of disillusionment and helplessness. She suggests the benefits of three things:

- Encouraging an inner journey, getting in touch with your soul
- Reflecting on beauty, noticing nature and the simple things in life, and
- Valuing justice and morality

Using art was effective in Simon's case. Other educative strategies or vehicles to assist exploration and expression of these things can include poetry, excerpts from biographies, personal testimonials, songs, mantras, affirmations, yoga, meditation and rituals. These can all function as conversation starters (McAllister *et al.*, 2004) and lead the way for the client to add cultural sources to their repertoire of coping resources.

Theory into Practice

On one level, Simon's story was an unusual tale because he was one of the few adolescents who actually do go on to receive professional mental health care. But on another level, his experience was common – he experienced changes he could not understand, he felt like he was not able to gain the support he needed, and felt pushed to an extreme so that he resorted to a severe incident of self-harm.

We know that young people underutilize many of the health services that are available to them, perhaps because of the associated stigma or simply due to lack of awareness of their existence (Gorman, Brough and Ramirez, 2003). When services are sought it is provided by General Practitioners and school-based counsellors. Of the youth who do access services, the best benefits are usually seen in help finding accommodation, employment and emotional support. Most young people are, however, more likely to seek support from those around them. But for Simon, who could find no one with whom he could talk in his family or school environments, mental health care was appropriate and effective.

Being Solution Oriented When Working with Young People

According to Stacey *et al.* (2002), all experienced youth workers, being an effective and solution-focused youth worker, means that we can:

- Respect young people as knowledgeable
- Respect different opinions
- Challenge ourselves to go beyond seeing young people as objects or people at risk. They have strengths and resilience
- Facilitate trust and listen with genuineness
- Acknowledge that partnerships do not always start from equal positions. There are some with more privilege and freedom to act on their power and they need to be accountable.
- Try to see solutions instead of just the problem, so look for the problem and then work on solutions.
- Focus on exceptions to the problem laden story so you can use those exceptions to build solutions
- Involve young people in as many aspects of the service as possible so, share decision making
- Try to see the problem as manageable by maintaining hope and optimism
- Attempt to find meaning during social interaction. Sometimes interactions can be educative and enlightening, rather than always simply fun or a distraction
- Change the way we look at a problem, because this will produce a change in future action and effects, so help the young person to describe their often-told stories differently
- Keep channels of communication open by maintaining conversation even when there may be silences and obstacles

Reader Activity: Within the story, a number of strategies of being solution focused were applied. Write down the content and rationale for the comments and questions that the nurse made in Simon's Story. How effective do you think the nurse was in joining with, building and extending Simon's skills? What other strategies could have been applied?

An important aim in working with someone like Simon who used self-harm as a coping strategy is to balance acceptance with change. Marsha Linehan (1993) in her work on Dialectical Behaviour Therapy explained that a major challenge for clients and clinicians is to understand that tension exists between the need to accept present coping mechanisms and obstacles, and the expectation that change will happen. This dialectic requires a kind of patient optimism. It is important to focus on being available, actively listening without judgment, encouraging him to talk, being willing to share some of one's own views, as well as share a concern for him with honesty. It may be frustrating sometimes because of a natural desire to intervene and fix problems, but it is important to encourage the young person to access their own resources and to see himself as a capable provider.

Managing Self-injury

Particularly distressing for many health care workers is this issue of deliberate self-injury. It is a fact that a common issue occurring in childhood is abuse and neglect. While there is no evidence that Simon had this experience, it needs to be explored. Conservative statistics estimate the incidence to be 3 in 1000 children (Angus and Woodward, 1995). But these are the cases of substantiated abuse. Many more cases go unreported or unrecorded and the figures are much higher in indigenous children. One in 10 of these children reported as abused or neglected in Australia are further abused within a year. One extreme way that young people sometimes use to express and manage memories of distress and ongoing feelings of inadequacy or confusion is to self-harm. Up to 30 per cent of those who self-harm are currently depressed (Hawton *et al.* 1998) and self-harm, while not synonymous with attempted suicide, is a risk factor for suicide. Therefore it is imperative that this action be taken seriously, and that clinicians use the best available evidence to guide their responses.

A number of key concepts helpful in understanding and responding to the young person who self-harms are as follows:

1. Begin by sifting out myth from reality (Table 7.1)
2. Remember that self-harm usually performs a protective or communicative function. The immediate aim is not to eliminate the behaviour, but to accept it as a coping strategy and work to find a safer alternative
3. Work with what's going right with the young person, focus on their uniqueness, their complexity and their hope
4. Facilitate their resilience
5. Use a framework (see Table 7.2) that helps you to plan the care proactively, rather than allowing you to react to problems or issues as they arise
6. If the person sees their self-harm in unhelpful, or damaging ways, work with them to try to reframe it (Table 7.3)

7. Explore, trial and select new coping mechanisms with the young person, such as learning to bear the moment rather than escape it, learning to moderate emotional extremes by using self-soothing and calming self-talk, being mindful rather than mindless.
8. Facilitate social connections with and for the young person, such as self-help groups and sporting and leisure groups where the person can find outlets or distraction from stressors
9. Provide opportunities for the person to be helpful and willing, rather than helpless and wilful
10. Invent and use strategies that help the young person realize that they are more than their problem, they have parts that are good, strong, resilient and unique, and together aim to enhance and develop them
11. Introduce meaning and ritual that helps the person mark their progress, so that they can notice small changes, achievements and so build hope.

Table 7.1 Myths of self-harm (McAllister, 2003)

True or False

1. Self-harm is always a symptom of severe personality disorder
2. Self-harm is the opposite of being suicidal
3. Hospitalization is the best practice for preventing further episodes of self-harm
4. 'Attention seeking behaviour' is the same as 'Acting out'
5. Nurses can't help someone who self-harms because his/her needs are too complex

Table 7.2 Reframing

Hunter and Chandler (1999) provide an interesting reframe of risk taking, self-destructive behaviours in young people as 'unhelpful resilience tactics'. Framed in this way, one begins to notice that Simon's tendency to isolate and disconnect himself from others, and to self-harm were also ways that he was signaling his strength and endurance. Using this notion, you could acknowledge and accept these behaviours, but also work to help him change. You could talk about resilience and the idea that some tactics are adaptive and others are unhelpful. Together you could make a list of tactics, labeled helpful and unhelpful and work to reframe them.

Helpful	**Unhelpful**
Willing	Willful
Determined	Stubborn
Self-soothe	Self-Harm
Assert	Yell
Cry	Cut
Run	Smoke

Resilience in a client can be promoted, even during times of crisis, by conveying optimism and faith in the person's ongoing capacity to cope. So, one can accept and also show the client another way to think about the issue or gently reframe negative self-talk so that he/she can see the self in new and more positive ways.

Conclusion

Being solution oriented in relation to young people, requires that we work towards a community that exists in partnership with young people, rather than in opposition or struggle. This chapter has discussed many ways of working with and for the young person and the community. Young people have a strength and an enthusiasm for life that can be contagious and invigorating and so youth work can be deeply rewarding. On the other hand, working with some of the tensions can be challenging. As we know from our knowledge of solution-focused approaches, there are various ways of expressing and managing this tension so that it works for us rather than against us. It is legitimate to be critical of the pressures that seem to be mounting for young people in today's world. But it is also important to have realistic expectations for change, and to continue to see the world as filled with possibilities.

Group Activity: The media frequently contains stories featuring young people. And usually television shows present young people in a positive, perhaps idealised light – it engages the young person, entertains, distracts and ultimately seduces them into buying products being advertised in the commercial breaks. But when young people are not the target audience for media stories, is adolescence portrayed in such flattering terms? A critical reading may be illuminating.

Select a local newspaper and analyse the content searching for the ways young people are represented. What ideas and values are being conveyed? Are there any myths or stereotypes that emerge? Are there any recurring themes?

Make a table, see the example below, comparing the qualitative, descriptive terms used to represent youth in film/television/magazine stories that you think are targeting youth with those that are targeting older adults. Critically analyse these major sources for understanding adolescence.

Quality (e.g. lazy, selfish, eager, helpful, reckless, smart)	**Representations of Youth**	
	Targetting youth	Targetting older adults

Suggestions for Further Reading

Alderman, T. (1997). *The scarred soul: Understanding and ending self-inflicted violence.* Oakland, CA: New Harbinger.

National Self-harm Network. *Hurt yourself less workbook.* London: Mental Health Foundation.

Shepperd, C. and McAllister, M. (2003). C.A.R.E: A framework for responding therapeutically to the client who self-harms. *Journal of Psychiatric and Mental Health Nursing, 10(4).* 442–447.

Slattery, P. (2001). *Youth works: A very practical book about working with young people.* Dulwich Hill, Australia: Peter Slattery.

Teacher notes to accompany this chapter can be found at www.palgrave.com/nursinghealth/mcallister

References

Angus, G. and Woodward, S. (1995). Child abuse and neglect Australia, 1993–94: *Australian Institute of Health and Welfare: Child Welfare Series No. 13.* Canberra: AGPS.

Bryan, B., and Batch, J. (2002). The complexities of ethnic adolescent health. *Youth Studies Australia, 21*(1), 24–33.

Burns, J., and Hickie, I. (2002). Depression in young people: A national school-based initiative for prevention, early intervention and pathways for care. *Australasian Psychiatry, 10*(2), 134–138.

Commonwealth Department of Health and Aged Care (2000). *MindMatters: A mental health promotion resource for secondary schools.* Mental Health and Special Programs Branch. Canberra: Commonwealth Department of Health and Aged Care.

Gorman, D., Brough, M. and Ramirez, E. (2003). How young people from culturally and linguistically *diverse backgrounds experience mental health: Some insights for mental health nurses. International Journal of Mental Health Nursing, 12*, 194–202.

Hawton, K., Arensman, E., Townsend, E. *et al.*, (1998). Deliberate self-harm: Systematic review of efficacy of psychosocial and pharmacological treatments in preventing repetition. *British Medical Journal, 31*, 441–447.

Hetherington, E. and Stanley-Hagan, M. (1999). The adjustment of children with divorced parents: A risk and resiliency perspective. *Journal of Child Psychology and psychiatry, 40*(1), 129–140.

Hunter, A., and Chandler, G. (1999). Adolescent resilience. *Image: Journal of Nursing Scholarship, 31*(3), 243–251.

Kang, M. (2002). Substance abuse in teenagers. Trends and consequences. *Australian Family Physician, 31* (1), 8–11.

Linehan, M. (1993). *Cognitive-behavioral treatment of borderline personality disorder.* New York: The Guilford Press.

McAllister, M. (2003). Self-harm in the Emergency Setting: Understanding and Responding. *Contemporary Nurse. 15* (1–2), 130–139.

McAllister, M., Matarasso, B., Dixon, B., and Shepperd, C. (2004). Conversation Starters: Reexamining and reconstructing first encounters within the therapeutic relationship. *Journal of Psychiatric and Mental Health Nursing*. 11, 575–582.

McAllister, M. and Walsh, K. (2003). C.A.R.E: A Framework for Mental Health Practice. *Journal of Psychiatric and Mental Health Nursing. 10*(1), 39–48.

McCann, I. and Pearlman, L. (1990). Vicarious traumatization: A framework for understanding the psychological effects of working with victims. *Journal of Traumatic Stress*, 3, 131–149.

Meadows, G. and Singh, B. (2001). *Mental health in Australia.* Oxford UP, Melbourne.

National Drug Research Institute (2001). *Community action helps to tackle drug use among young people.* Accessed on the world wide web on 27 June, 2004 at www.curtin.edu.au/curtin/centre/ndri/news/media/2001.

Rapp, C. (1989). The strengths model of case management: Results from twelve demonstrations. *Psychosocial Rehabilitation Journal. 13*(1), 23–31.

Ritzer, G. (1993). *The McDonaldization of society: An investigation into the changing character of contemporary social life.* Thousand Oaks, CA: Pine Forge Press.

Sanders, M., Tully, L., Turner, K., Maher, C., and McAuliffe, C. (2003). Training GPs in parent consultation skills. An evaluation of training for the Triple P-Positive Parenting Program. Australian Family Physician, *32*(9), 763–768.

Sawyer, M., Arney, F., Baghurst, P., Clark, J., Graetz, B., Kosky, R., Nurcombe, B., Patton, G., Prior, M., Raphael, B., Rey, J., Whaites, L., and Zubrick, S. (2000). The mental health of young people in Australia: The child and adolescent component of the national survey of mental health and wellbeing. Canberra: Ausinfo.

Stacey, K., Webb, E., Hills, S., Lagzdins, N., Moulds, D., Phillips, T. and Stone, P. (2002). Relationships and power. *Youth Studies Australia, 21*(1), 44–51.

Webber, R. (2002). Young people and their quest for meaning. *Youth Studies Australia, 21*(1), 40–43.

Welton, M. (1995). *In defense of the lifeworld. Critical perspectives on adult learning.* New York: State University of New York Press.

CHAPTER 8

Expanding Nurses' Capabilities in Acute Care

Amanda Henderson

Overview

This chapter explores how solution focused nursing can expand nurses' understanding of and responses to patients' experiences in the alien environment of the acute care setting. Acute care knowledge has developed in parallel with the growth in medical knowledge, which also saw the development of the hospital system. As you will see, particular norms and dominant ideologies have become synonymous with this way of organizing health care. These have had a significant influence on how health care is understood and supported by nursing. Patients' stories are a powerful way of revealing how these norms and dominant ideologies influence health care experiences. This chapter presents 'snapshots' of patients in the acute care situation. It explores the contingencies of these snapshots and encourages the reader to empathize with and analyse how patients may interpret their episode of acute illness. Solution focused nursing is an approach that helps nurses take apart the contingencies of acute care in order to progress patients towards health outcomes relevant to long term well-being.

The Development of Medical Knowledge

Acute care has largely been attended in the domain of the hospital. Hospitals have had no continuous evolution however their form corresponds to the peculiar features of the society in which they have become embedded (Turner, 1995). Therefore how society views health and illness, will give insight into why and how acute care services are arranged in the way that they are.

During the nineteenth century, physicians developed and refined a series of instruments and techniques of bodily manipulation, which located and identified the place of illness and the lesion that produced it (Aronowitz, 1998). This new perspective in diagnosing and treating health conditions resulted in a new kind of doctor-patient interaction. No longer were interactions centred on the patient's experience of illness – particularly the symptoms they were suffering – but rather on diagnostic procedures. The confounding factor is that doctors 'are fascinated with disembodied anatomic realities, even when we have substantial reason to believe that they relate less and less to what bothers our patients or what ultimately happens to our patients' (Baron, 1985, p. 607).

As we read in Chapter 2, for a long time health care was shaped almost exclusively by an empirical view of the world. Medical ideology emerged from that world view and has been summarized by Waitzkin (1983, pp. 56–57) as emphasising:

- Disturbances of biological homeostasis are equivalent to breakdown of machines
- Disease is a problem of the individual human being
- Science permits the rational control of human beings
- Many spheres of life are appropriate for medical management
- Medical science is both esoteric and excellent

These ideas form the basis of the traditional doctor-patient interaction. In this interaction, typically the patient presents to the doctor in the belief that their health problem is because 'something has gone wrong in their body'. The doctor, through investigative tests and procedures, is able to 'locate' the problem and appropriately intervene to 'fix' the problem.

The Evolution of the Hospital

This view of illness has been reinforced and indeed institutionalized, through the organization of care. A later historical development, the appearance of hospitals, is allied to the growth of 'scientific inquiry'. The hospital came about initially as a residence for poor and invalid people: wealthy people were generally treated in their own homes. However, with specialization of services, individuals were no longer routinely treated in their own homes, but in an institution – namely the hospital – which permitted resources to be collected in one area (Bullough and Bullough, 1972, p. 94).

Although a medieval development, hospitals gradually shifted their focus in the eighteenth century, from poor houses to institutions that taught clinical medicine, as physicians started recognising their potential for greater observation and monitoring. With the growth of scientific medicine, it became convenient and efficient for doctors to place sick people in a building where doctors and nurses could care for groups of patients (Nyberg, 1991, p. 245) and similarly the collection of exact facts about patients' condition could be organized. The clustering of those patients with like signs and symptoms together reinforced the reification of disease and led to specialization by disease or body area.

Specialization was seen by the medical profession as necessary to improve modern medical practice and so a considerable proportion of all physicians limited their work to one field (Rosen, 1972). This resulted in further increases in the number and size of hospitals, as patients were further encouraged to attend hospital rather than be cared for in their own home. However, while supposedly more successful in separating specific illnesses so that specialized treatment can be administered, specialization means that any client might be seen by a number of medical specialists, contributing to the social distancing of doctors from the patient (Turner, 1995).

In today's society, hospitals have assumed a highly significant position and are of symbolic importance as central institutions of goodwill (Daniel, 1990). 'Their antecedents had been dreaded, ugly repositories for the insane and diseased, but modern hospitals serve entirely different functions and are dedicated to medical science and humanitarian values' (Daniel, 1990, p. 67). In support, Turner (1995) argues that the expansion of medical knowledge and its legitimacy in turn have accompanied the contemporary growth and specialization of hospitals as the principal settings of medical technology and practice.

Individuals have an expectation of high quality of life and they expect that health care providers within the institution can help them achieve this goal (Cramer and Tucker, 1995). As hospitals are the focus of highly esteemed medical practices it is the expectation that individuals will receive the best possible care when in hospital. Hence the hospital has come to occupy a powerful symbolic place in modern health care. People tend to view the hospital as a place where they will be given appropriate care, and where health problems will be solved.

The treatment of health problems is also known as secondary prevention because early, effective treatment is important in the prevention of chronic disease and disability that can develop when an illness is not treated promptly. It is widely recognized that secondary prevention is one part in a three part process of comprehensive health care. Primary and tertiary prevention programs are also important. Primary prevention is of course the prevention of an illness from occurring in the first place. Vaccination is an example of primary prevention. Tertiary prevention is the application of rehabilitation principles in order to reduce the impact that a chronic or ongoing condition has on a person's life functioning and ability. Vocational and lifestyle support programs are examples. All three have an important role to play.

However, because of the power of medical and scientific knowledge to set the agenda in health care policy and reform, it is this secondary prevention model, and the growth of hospital services and diagnostic and treatment services, that has been allowed to flourish. Thus, one can appreciate that the hospital has a valuable place, but its primacy indeed, its omnipotence, can at times create tension and lead to silences and gaps in social and community services.

Reader Activity: Recall when you first entered a large hospital or health service. How did it differ from other environments with which you were familiar? In particular, reflect on architectural and design aspects. What elements do you believe give it symbolic power? Do you believe that these features influence interactions in the environment?

The Influence of Science in the Practice of Caring for Patients

Such institutional factors shaped by society are instrumental in firming the establishment of scientific knowledge in everyday practice (Wynne, 1991, p. 116). Scientific knowledge 'comes clothed in social and institutional forms and cannot easily be divorced from those associated social prescriptions, interests and orientations' (Wynne, 1991, p. 115). While Wynne (1991) refers to scientific knowledge throughout many aspects of our society this notion is of particular relevance to acute health care as it is practised in hospitals. Wynne emphasizes that 'these structures may not be deliberately chosen by scientists but may nevertheless be structured into the knowledge central to these disciplines, for example, via the questions that are emphasized, the degree of standardisation that is imposed, or the extent to which uncertainties are withheld (even for the best of reasons)' (p. 116).

This situation has implications for how patients understand and experience their acute episodes of care as well as how nurses respond. It is scientific knowledge, and the valuing of categorization, that influences how patients are allocated to different wards in highly specialized hospitals. For example, when patients are admitted to a surgical ward then the focus of health care (and thus for nursing care) is the preparation of the patient for medical/surgical intervention, the provision of assistance with the implementation of the intervention, followed by post-operative care. Accompanying medical issues, psycho-social concerns, or broadening understanding of the situation that the patient now finds themselves are generally given little recognition (Henderson, 2005). Dominant ideology has a powerful yet subtle influence over health care practitioners, it shapes and constrains clinicians' practices. Thus, whilst many nurses may have been trained to be concerned for a client's personal, cultural and unique needs and to be proactive by educating clients about lifestyle and health management, in acute care settings such as hospitals nurses can be so heavily influenced by the prevailing medical/scientific ideology that their role is reduced to medical care and medical assistance work.

Reader Activity: Think about acute care services that you or your family have experienced and use this to answer the following questions:

- How would you describe the typical acute care nurse's role?

When nurses interacted with you, what kinds of questions were commonly asked?

> Compare and contrast the concerns of scientific knowledge and the way a hospital is run, with the concerns of nursing knowledge.
>
> - What kinds of standardizations can you recall?
> - What uncertainties were withheld and why?
> - What were the effects?

An understanding based on scientific rigour facilitates the development of standardized policies and procedures. Such standardization is important as it ensures minimum standards through stipulating the steps of a procedure and encouraging the practitioner to check the actions based on these steps. The increasing use of standard policies and procedures has been beneficial in guiding and ensuring standards for clinical activities that occur across a large complex health care system with at times, different staff with different backgrounds and experience. Arguably standardization contributes to safe and cost-effective care. More recently there is a push to further ground these guidelines in evidence, usually research based, to justify their effectiveness. It is important to note that even in the case of evidence based guidelines, nursing practice delivered to any client is about providing for their unique situation. Nurses need to understand patients' specific situation and within the context of guidelines provide nursing care to maximize the benefits of their health care interventions.

For busy nurses, it can sometimes be tempting to apply standardized procedures to all patients. Routines can provide predictability and can assist in the smooth functioning of complicated workplaces. However, it is also possible to be efficient, scientific, diligent and controlled whilst also being sensitive, humane and caring as this next story illustrates.

An Acute Care Story: Anne and Jane

Jane is a first year RN working the evening shift in an acute medical ward at a major hospital. She's about to answer the buzzer of a patient she has not yet met, so she quickly consults the Unit board – Bed 16 C: Anne Brown, 65 years, Leg Ulcer for OT in the am.

Anne, lying awkwardly across her bed, is visibly upset and moaning softly. She is so tired, it's been a very long day. At 6 am she and her husband rose to have an early breakfast so that they could make their way through traffic to the busy city hospital for their 9 am appointment. Arriving on time they sat down to wait. Two hours went by before she was ushered in to another waiting area until eventually she saw a Doctor. The news was not good, she had to be admitted because her ulcer was infected and slow to heal. She was told she'd need antibiotics and the wound surgically cleaned. So she was in for another wait, while a bed was found. It wasn't until 5 pm that she was taken to a ward, allocated a bed and able to sip her first cup of tea for the day.

All Anne wants to do now is rest, but in this brightly lit, austere room she knows she will never sleep. It's not like home – a comfy little cottage in a leafy quiet suburb on the outskirts of town. A dull ache in her chest has not gone away and now she is getting worried. She doesn't want to bother the nurses, she knows they are constantly running to attend to sicker people than she, but right now, she just doesn't know what to do. What is this pain? It doesn't feel right.

Jane enters the room and quickly sees that Anne needs assistance. She is sweating, grimacing, she appears to be in pain. Jane states quietly and confidently that she will help Anne to move into a more comfortable position and requests that she be permitted to take a full set of observations. These are completed and show that Anne is moderately tachycardic, hypertensive and hypoxic. Jane is also concerned about Anne's pain and so asks a series of questions to explore the nature, position and duration of the pain. She learns that Anne is having centralized chest-pain, that four years ago she was diagnosed with Angina. For this Anne applies an Anginine patch for 12 hours daily – only this morning, in all the rush to get to the wound clinic, Anne forgot to put it on and three hours ago she began to feel a tightness and now this gripping pain.

Jane completes the physical health assessment, recording the data in the bedside chart. She has a plan in her head: Anne will probably need supplemented Oxygen, an ECG and sublingual Anginine Stat, and it is therefore important to contact the medical team as soon as possible.

But Jane is also quite aware that Anne is anxious and tired and knows that this can make chest pain worse. Jane also makes a mental note to speak with the nurse consultant about long term strategies to enhance comfort for all patients such as Anne should they need to endure long waiting periods. Jane turns once again to Anne, speaking quietly, confidently, but with a slower more reassuring tone …

'Mrs Brown, I think with the stress of this long day and not having your usual medication your Angina has recurred. It's also no wonder that you're tired and upset. I think that what we should do is contact the doctor immediately so that we can recommence medication and check your heart more closely. Do you agree?' Anne nods and takes Jane's hand in gratitude.

Jane continues soothingly, 'and in the meantime you and I could work together on ways to make you more comfortable. Have you found that relaxing, breathing deeply and settling down can help your pulse slow and your pain ease?'

Reader Activity: A dominant scientific ideology in the acute care environment is characterized by a focus on medical/surgical intervention.

- In what ways does the nurse in this story support this ideology?

In what ways does she move beyond this ideology towards being solution focused?

Analyse the interaction that takes place between Anne and Jane and find examples that appraise how well Jane implements the joining, building and extending phases of SFN?
SFN is concerned not just with personal patient care, but also with creating change in the interests of social justice. What issues arise that indicate Jane's concern for social well-being?

Nurses, because of their training, familiarity and proximity to scientific and medical knowledge are likely to know far more about health issues than acute care clients. But this doesn't mean that clients have no wisdom or expert knowledge. Yet sometimes, the very position within the dynamic of nurse-patient can give and take away the power that usually comes with knowledge. In the acute care setting, the nurse is frequently positioned as the expert and yet sometimes may be naïve and unknowing (Jane is a first year RN and thus there is likely to be much that she does not yet understand). At the same time, the patient is frequently positioned as lacking expertise, regardless of their background or familiarity with the health problem. For example, medications are routinely removed from patients, and patients are required to wait and be passive whilst interventions are performed 'on' their bodies. This is one of the negative consequences of a scientifically-controlled health care system.

How Practice Shapes What We Know and Do Not Know

Not only are patients influenced by the routine practices of doctors and other health professionals in this acute care context who subtly, and sometimes not so subtly indicate that scientific and medical knowledge as well as the efficient running of the system must come before human needs, but so too is knowledge development.

Practices that are based in scientific knowledge, tend to be instrumental in the development of patients' understanding of their health. Not surprisingly then, patients frequently come to value and only value aspects about health and illness that are defined scientifically, or supported medically.

Reader Activity: Reflect for a moment on the WHO definition of health.
Health is a state of complete physical, mental and social well-being and not merely the absence of disease or infirmity.
Yet, the practical objective of most acute care hospital units is to achieve absence of disease or infirmity.

- What do you suggest nurses could contribute so that Acute Care Units work to achieve the WHO definition of health?

Rouse (1987) made the distinction that we should not only understand the authority of scientific achievement by what is 'known', but we also need to investigate 'how the natural sciences have changed us and in what terms we can critically understand and assess these changes' (p. x). If we are to adopt this premise, our specific interest is not what scientific knowledge has been able to explain, prove, demonstrate or predict, but rather how such knowledge operates in the hospital environment, how this interrelates with 'everyday' commonsense knowledge and its impact on both patient and doctor in terms of reaching the desired outcome for the patient.

Rouse suggests that, because the acquisition of scientific knowledge requires the careful observation and monitoring of events, this in itself transforms the 'field of possible action', thereby shaping practices and knowledge (p. 240). Rouse's concern is to decipher how such practices influence the development of knowledge.

An example of this is the nurse working in intensive care who observes the physiological parameters of the patient in intensive care, yet does not read the emotional status of the patient as precisely (Henderson, 1994).

Rouse advocates a critical understanding of the domination of scientific knowledge. He states that this is not because 'science should be rejected, abandoned or even necessarily modified in significant ways (if it were even possible, let alone desirable, to abandon science in a society in which it is so intertwined with other practices)' (Rouse, 1987, p. 208) but rather the aim of his criticism is to *situate* the sciences within the configuration of practices that shape our shared possibilities today in order to provide a better understanding of our situation (Rouse, 1987, p. 208).

Interpretation is a matter of coming to see what is 'at issue' in how someone lives – that is, not the causes, but rather how and why these causes have come to be significant (Rouse, 1987, p. 48). This is particularly relevant to patients in the acute context who acknowledge that the doctor knows all about the 'science' of their condition however, patients want doctors to understand what they are experiencing and assist them in the management of these experiences (Lacroix, Jacquemet and Assal, 1995). In relation to the acute health care setting, patients have stated that they do not necessarily desire extensive information about what is happening at a cellular or even systems level in the body but rather they have expressed a desire for doctors to understand what it is like for the patient to 'live' with the disease or condition (Lacriox, Jacquemet and Assal, 1995). This request for information has arisen from patients living with chronic conditions. Their experience with their disease has resulted in their ability to clearly articulate their needs. The concern for many patients in the acute context is that often they are experiencing an episode for the first time and therefore may not have sufficient insight or experience to ask the questions which are most meaningful to their everyday lifestyle (Henderson, 2006).

Implications for Patients' Impressions and Expectations of Health Care

Shirley's Story

Shirley was admitted to the medical ward via the Coronary Care Unit (CCU). Whilst she had had a lot of prior experience with hospitalization, since her heart had been functioning poorly for many years, Shirley was anxious and distressed. The medical team acted quickly to provide her with information that they hoped would alleviate her worry.

The consultant doctor explained to her that she had a 'murmur'. He drew a diagram showing her how the valves in her heart were not operating effectively and how her body needed time to repair. This explanation rested comfortably with her – she believed she understood it, and Shirley's anxiety and distress quickly dissipated. She also believed she was able to comply with the doctor's instructions readily because she now had an understanding of what was happening to her.

After admission Shirley was prescribed bed rest. This made sense for her because Shirley felt particularly lethargic. She was also well aware of the reduced functioning capacity of her heart. She described her heart as 'precarious' and therefore had to 'take care with it'.

Another requirement for Shirley's care was to be hospitalized so that she could be observed and scientific information obtained about the functional capacity of her body. Nurses regularly monitored her vital signs such as, pulse rate, blood pressure, respirations and ECG. Blood tests and X-rays were also conducted to provide further information about electrolytes and fluid status.

Shirley progressively mobilized out of bed after her period of confinement. Within three days she was able to be assisted to the shower. Shirley asked many questions of the medical team, but often doctors were too busy to provide complete information and sometimes Shirley felt self-conscious about taking up too much of their time. Nonetheless, Shirley was feeling better and more able to be self-caring. However, at this stage and without explanation, Shirley was moved from near the sister's station to a single room, away from the central activity area.

Having previously been told that she needed to be under constant observation and monitoring, Shirley felt confused, ignored and abandoned. Since Shirley understood hospital care to be about the conduct of tests and observations of functioning, and that she now had confidence in her own capacity to self-care, she could see no value in being in hospital and was no longer happy to be in acute care and Shirley requested discharge.

Important Themes within Shirley's Story

Although Shirley had been admitted to hospital on many occasions before and was aware of the regime, she still felt anxious with her sudden physical deterioration. This is an important time for nurses to provide assertive, reassuring support and to focus on the extending phase of solution focused nursing. In this phase, the intensive support provided in the earlier phases of the relationship can be expected to be gradually reduced. Also, the skills acquired and developed within the building phase are encouraged to be practised with less supervision and more independence. When the extending phase is noticed, valued and used, one might expect that the client experiences less of a sense of abandonment, and more a sense of accomplishment. Upon reflection, perhaps the extending phase deserved greater focus.

Shirley understood the reason for her admission to acute care was for her condition to be monitored. At first Shirley had complete faith in what was explained and consequently was happy to adhere to instructions and to stay in hospital. But soon, Shirley also began to appreciate her own role in self-care and that she needed more information. However, such self-awareness was not encouraged in the hospital environment, where medical control and diagnosis tends to take precedence over patient-control and patient knowledge.

When sufficient diagnostic procedures had been completed, Shirley was moved to an area remote from the sister's station and the general activity of the ward. To Shirley, this was an important transition time, but the health care team unfortunately routinised the move and failed to notice or act on its significance for Shirley.

There are many important characters in this story, not the least is the part played by the Acute Care Nurse. Not much, however, has been said about what nurses did, or could have done, whilst working with Shirley.

Reader Activity: 1. Linked to the notion of the extending phase is the role of transition worker. Revise your understanding of nurses as transition worker, explained in Chapters 1and 3.

2. Identify critical moments in this story, where nurses could have played a supportive, educative and facilitative role.
3. Identify issues that would assist Shirley to make a successful transition from acute care to independent living.

Relate the answers you provided to some of the principles and concepts I consider to be important to acute care nursing.

1. Nurses with advanced skills in acute care are those who can merge technical knowledge and skills of medical management with interpersonal skills.
2. Empathy and support can be provided, by way of non-verbal communication, use of touch, space and support, throughout the delivery of even the most complex medical procedure.

3. Emotional support is positively correlated with healing and recovery. Support may promote catharsis, releasing fears, anger, frustration, or helplessness that might otherwise be suppressed and accumulated to later delay recovery.
4. In situations where clients become distressed, nurses can help them to reframe a negative viewpoint into something that is positive and more manageable. For example, in this experience Shirley might look upon the move to a room further away from the sister's office, not as evidence of abandonment, but as evidence of growing independence, a challenge for self-care.
5. The role of transition is most apparent when an acute health problem begins to resolve. When nurses are present to facilitate that transition they can normalize the transfer home. They may encourage the client to reflect on their hospitalization as a positive experience and ultimately learn from it. Important in this process is asking questions, listening, being there to respond to the client's questions and comments.
6. Health Education in acute care involves assessing the patient's knowledge of the illness, readiness to learn and the lifestyle they desire. It involves provision of practical information and follow up resources, triggering issues rather than overloading the person with content knowledge.

Exploring Solutions within the Domain of the Acute Setting

Practices within the acute care setting are very influential in how patients interpret and understand their health. In interactions with patients, nurses have an opportunity to re-focus these practices so that they are supportive of patients' attempts to be discerning health care consumers, and well informed self-carers. Solution focused nursing will only successfully emerge in the acute care context when 'science' is successfully situated as just one aspect of care provisions and other dimensions of patient care are given a voice.

Nurses can facilitate solution focused nursing through honest and clear discussion and communication about the end points of care. This honest communication is not so much about explaining *what* the procedure involves, but rather negotiating the different end points that each individual wants and some form of agreement whereby there is a realistic assessment of the degree to which these can be met. Assistance is needed to encourage and help patients articulate their knowledge; to help them see the value of their experiences, feelings and sensations. Nurses have a responsibility to foster this development of patient knowledge.

Nurses need to encourage dialogue with patients about: What is important in their lives; What particular resolution they would like in this acute episode; What is a realistic and achievable situation. It may involve nurses drawing on the services of other professionals for psychological assistance or assistance through physical aids with life style when they return home.

Essentially, a repositioning of knowledge is required. The public need to be re-educated to understand that scientific knowledge is just one aspect of their health care. Other domains of knowledge need to be articulated and made known through different methods of communication, for example, patients should not just be passive recipients of information of tests. Patients' experiences, understanding and concerns should be an integral concern for nurses, to ensure that there is an appropriate response to their needs.

Such a move would fit with Wynne's (1991) proposal for scientific institutions to relate to public agendas and consequently develop a greater level of trust with the public. Wynne advocates that, to assist with intersubjective understanding and attain a level of trust, scientific institutions 'must be organized so as to better understand and relate to public agendas and knowledge, rather than appear to wish to impose a scientific (which often means, standardized) framework of understanding as if that on its own were adequate' (p. 115).

Conclusion

Knowledge development in the scientific domain has considerable implications for how health is known and understood. The importance of experience, feeling, emotion and interpretation are largely subjugated (Turner, 1995). If contemporary health care is to continue to provide a satisfactory service to provide for the needs of an educated and more active community then it is essential that service providers engage in a mutually satisfactory relationship with their clients. It is imperative that nurses as a major provider within health services engender a sense of trust and mutual co-operation in the population that they are serving.

Suggestions for Further Reading

Henderson, A. (1994). Power and knowledge in nursing practice: the contribution of Foucault. *Journal of Advanced Nursing*, *20*(5), 935–939.

References

Aronowitz, R. (1998). *Making sense of Illness.* United Kingdom: Cambridge University Press.

Baron, R. (1985). An introduction to medical phenomenology: I can't hear you while I'm listening. *Annals of Internal Medicine, 103*, 606–611.

Bullough, B. and Bullough, V. (1972). A brief history of medical practice. In E. Freidson and J. Lorber (eds), *Medical men and their work* (pp. 86–102). Chicago: Aldine Atherton.

Cramer, D. and Tucker, S. (1995). The consumer's role in quality: partnering for quality outcomes. *Journal of Nursing Care Quality, 9*(2), 54–66.

Daniel, A. (1990). *Medicine and the state.* Sydney: Allen and Unwin.
Henderson, A. (2006). Boundaries around the 'well-informed' patient: the contribution of Schutz to inform nurses' interactions. *Journal of Clinical Nursing. 15*, 4–10.
Lacroix, A., Jacquemet, S. and Assal, J. (1995). Patients' experiences with their disease: learning from the differences and sharing the common problems. *Patient Education and Counseling, 26*, 301–312.
Nyberg, J. (1991). The nurse as professnocrat. *Nursing Economics, 9*(4), 244–247.
Rosen, G. (1972). Changing Attitudes of the Medical Profession to Specialization. In E. Freidson and J. Lorber (eds), *Medical men and their work.* Chicago: Aldine Atherton.
Rouse, J. (1987). *Knowledge and power.* New York: Cornell University Press.
Turner, B (1995). *Medical power and social knowledge (2nd ed).* London: Sage.
Waitzkin, H. (1983). *The second sickness.* London: Collier Macmillan Publishers.
Wynne, B. (1991). Knowledges in context. *Science, Technology, and Human Values, 16*(1), 111–121.

CHAPTER 9

Solution Focused Mental Health Nursing

Kenneth Walsh and Cheryle Moss

Overview

There are various models for understanding mental disorders and their treatment, and it is possible to track their application across time. The psychodynamic model emerged in the early 20th century, followed by the medical model in the 1950s, the behavioural model in the 1960s, the humanistic model in the 1970s and the strengths model in the 1980s. Arguably the medical model has gained dominance in mainstream psychiatry, so that, despite the rhetoric of focusing on 'mental health', acute mental health services continue to prioritise treatment for serious mental illnesses such as Schizophrenia and Depression and inpatient care mainly involves assessment, containment and psychotropic medication administration. Emphasis on outcomes in mental health and medical management does not fit neatly with Mental Health Nursing values which have long focused on processes of care such as being human and building relationship. Such aspects of care are important to the process of health care delivery but much of it is difficult to measure. Indeed, qualities of kindness, patience, faith, compassion and hopefulness are immeasurable, but crucial to mental health nursing. This chapter critiques the preoccupations with outcomes of care arguing for a refocus to process, and shows how the process of being solution focused in mental health care is important, valuable and necessary for health and social services.

Peter's Story

Peter had suffered from Schizophrenia for many years and was now living and working in the community. Peter had built up a good relationship with staff of a School of Nursing and would help out each year by volunteering to participate in a mental status examination with Dave, a staff member of the School. The aim of the interview was to demonstrate interview techniques and was conducted in an interview room with students observing through a one-way mirror in an adjacent room. The interview progressed as normal and Peter spoke of his auditory hallucinations and his delusions. None of this was new to Dave until Peter stated that he believed that this year at Easter (about 4 weeks away) he would die. Peter explained that as he was the reincarnation of Jesus Christ and as he was now 33 and Christ died at Easter at the age of 33 then God would take his life at Easter. When Dave asked what would happen if God didn't take Peter's life at Easter, Peter replied that this would be a sign to him that he would have to take his own life.

Peter and Dave wrapped up the interview and following a review of risk, Peter and Dave agreed to meet the next morning for a follow up session together at Peter's flat. That evening Dave mused on how frightening it would be to be in Peter's situation. Peter believed himself to be in a 'Catch 22'. If he didn't die he would have to kill himself. The next morning Dave went to Peter's flat. Peter looked frightened. Dave spent some time talking with Peter about how he was feeling and together they outlined the background and the history of Peter's current circumstances. Peter had suffered from auditory hallucinations and delusions of varying intensity and content for many years. From time to time he had been hospitalized. He had been living independently for some years now and working in muffler repair shop.

Right now though, Peter was frightened because he didn't want to die. But if it really was God's will then what was he to do? There seemed to be a hint of doubt in Peter's voice. Were there times when he doubted it was God's will? Yes there were. Dave asked Peter to scale how strongly he believed that he was the reincarnation of Jesus Christ and would have to die, ten being he had no doubts and one being he doubted it very much. Peter scaled it at eight. Dave asked how strong his belief had been yesterday? Peter said it was more like ten yesterday. So what made the difference? Peter thought it was being able to talk about it with someone he trusted. He had long ago learnt to keep his beliefs to himself, especially around his work colleagues in the muffler repair shop. Peter was already looking more animated and relaxed. Dave and Peter agreed to have regular contact over the next few weeks. They also discussed the goals they would like to achieve together in this time. Peter said he would like to feel safe and not die.

At the next session Peter's assessment of his situation was that he felt about the same. Dave asked 'how come things aren't worse – what have you done to stop things from getting worse?' Peter thought it was because he had decided to tell Dave about his problem and do something about it. Dave then asked Peter that if by some chance a miracle happened and tomorrow he woke up and the problem was gone how would he know? Peter replied 'the voices would not be in my head and I would not feel so frightened'. Dave asked if there were times when this was already happening. Peter said there were times when he was bothered less by these thoughts and the voices. These times usually coincided with being around people he liked and being busy. Peter agreed to increase the amount of time he spent with friends at those times he felt most bothered by the voices (most commonly the weekends). He also identified activities he enjoyed and agreed to increase these activities in the immediate future.

Dave and Peter continued to work together on the puzzle of Peter's belief's and fears. They increased their contact with each other in the weeks leading up to Easter and Peter started to see his disturbing thoughts as a product of his illness. They tried out many solutions, some simple and some more complex such as Peter imagining he had a volume switch like on his radio so that he could turn the troublesome voices down. Peter and Dave worked with Peter's doctor to review his medication and just before Easter Peter asked to be admitted to the inpatient unit where he spent a safe and uneventful Easter.

Peter still lives in the community and still helps out with the student teaching activities of the school. Dave and he still work together on Peter's puzzles. Peter is building quite an armamentarium of solutions which he uses to cope with the peaks, troughs and transitions of his mental health.

Working Together Through a Mental Health Transition

Religious delusions such as those suffered by Peter, although somewhat clichéd, are not uncommon. Peter and Dave's story is an ordinary one, familiar to many mental health nurses and clients. Nevertheless it illustrates some key points that are important when working in a solution focused way. We use the term 'solution focussed way' deliberately here. There is a temptation to see SFN as a group of techniques which can be used to get a particular outcome (Lipchik, 2002). To do so is to miss the point of SFN. SFN is as much a way of comporting oneself with a client as it is a group of techniques. Today there is a tendency in society to go for the quick fix, be it in relation to diets, food preparation, treatment for illness, change management or counselling. This quick fix often revolves around instrumental solutions to problems sometimes devoid of contextual considerations (Saul, 2001). Solution-Focused Nursing, whilst it offers some techniques derived from solution focused counselling, takes place in the context of a nurse-patient relationship where techniques and the therapeutic encounter meet.

Therapeutic Alliance

The encounter between Peter and Dave took place in the context of an existing therapeutic relationship. Peter and Dave reflected on how Peter was feeling and they took their time to understand what was happening now in Peter's life and what he wanted to achieve. SFN is relationship driven not technique driven. A broad understanding of where the person's current mental health transition lies in relation to the person's life and what the person wants to achieve is important if multiple blind alleys are to be avoided. It was also important for Peter to develop trust in the relationship with Dave. This trust allayed his anxiety and helped him move to a position where he was more willing to explore solutions with Dave. Dave similarly needed to have a positive view of Peter's strengths. This cannot be understated. Miller and Rollnick (2002) who originated Motivational Enhancement Therapy, which shares some principles with SFN (Lewis and Osborn, 2004), state that the belief in the client's ability to change becomes a self-fulfilling prophecy. And like Motivational Enhancement, nursing in a solution focused way means that we listen rather than tell, seek to build up rather than tear down and to compliment rather than denigrate (Lewis and Osborn, 2004; Miller and Rollnick, 2002).

More Than Technique

Dave went on to use some of the techniques of SFN now familiar to readers. Specifically he used the scaling question and the miracle question (Quick, 1996; Lipchik, 2002; Webster, Vaughn and Martinez, 1994). See Table 9.1 for a list on commonly used solution-focused questions. Once again the context is as important as the content. The context of using the techniques was that they were used as tools to help the client focus on solutions and strengths. Regarding the latter Dave helped Peter reframe his situation in terms of what he was doing to stop things from getting worse. Again, in solutions focused therapy, as well as solution focused nursing, there can be a tendency to emphasize technique (Lipchik, 2002). This recipe focus is tantamount to teaching cooking by emphasizing the qualities of the non-stick fry pan and as we know, simply purchasing Teflon-ware does not create a good cook (more is the pity). Thus, it is unlikely that the scaling question in the absence of a strong therapeutic alliance, would elicit the client's doubts in the veracity of his beliefs. However, it is also worth mentioning that building a strong therapeutic alliance does not necessarily take a long time. Once again it is linked to the qualities of the therapeutic encounter. Some years back I (KW) encountered a

Table 9.1 Solution-Focused Nursing questions (Lipchik, 2002; Webster *et al.*, 1990)

What changes have you already noticed?
How would you know things were better … ?
Are there times when you already … ?
If you go to bed tonight and a miracle happens while you re asleep and when you wake up in the morning your problem is solved, how would things be different?
Tell me about those times when this problem doesn't occur. How do you get that to happen?
Does that already happen at times?
What will you have to do to make that happen?
What will have to happen for more of that to happen?
What could others do to help you?
How have you dealt with … … . in the past?
When you felt better a while ago what was different then?
How come things aren't worse – what have you done to stop things from getting worse?
On a scale of 1–10 with one being … and 10 being … tell me …

client I had worked with for one, two hour session twelve years previously. He believed the session had helped him by building hope at a time in his life when he had felt most vulnerable in his mental health transition. After twelve years he still remembered my name and could recount details of our encounter.

Another issue related to a focus on technique is that not all the techniques of SFN are applicable to every situation and some work better with some people than others. In the case study above, Peter, despite his experience of hallucinations and delusions, found the miracle question useful. This is not always the case and where technique is the major emphasis there may be a tendency on the part of the nurse to focus on the technique as a solution. Patients who do not benefit from a particular technique may pick up on the nurse's frustration and feel that in some way they have failed. Instead of building the self-esteem and self-efficacy, which may assist with their current circumstances, these qualities may in fact be diminished. So in working in nursing in a solution focused way, the process is as important as the outcome. Finding ways of working with clients that work for them is not a waste of time.

Understanding in SFN

So it is that in human to human encounters an appreciation of the humanity of the other is extremely valuable and will contribute to the efficacy of any techniques we employ. Through our appreciation of our shared humanity we can come to an understanding of the other person (Walsh, 1999). This is not as simple as it at first seems. An appreciation of the other person fundamentally more similar to us than different but nevertheless grounded in their individuality, is not easy. This is perhaps especially true when the person is suffering from a severe mental health transition. Partly this is because of the emphasis usually placed on diagnostic categories. Though classification systems offer some benefits they can, through their focus on lists of symptoms, blind us to the humanity of the other. It is perhaps easy to identify with and empathize with someone suffering from cancer. We can for the most part see ourselves in their position. However, few people can place themselves in the shoes of someone suffering from a severe mental health problem such as Schizophrenia. Yet the experience of mental health transition is understandable and people suffering from mental health transitions can be understood. Dave may not have experienced hallucinations or understood Peter's delusions but he could understand the very human reactions of fear, confusion and anxiety that stemmed from these. This appreciation of the humanity of the other can guide us when the other person's experience seems to bear no resemblance to our own.

Imagination in SFN

Partly this requires an appreciation of and an ability to use, imagination. Imagination has tended to get a bad press. We tend to view imagination in a pejorative way. We say, 'you are imagining things', 'don't let your imagination carry you away'. Yet imagination is the key to empathy and engagement and these in turn are the key to a strong therapeutic alliance. In discussing imagination and its role in medicine, the Canadian philosopher John Ralston Saul states that imagination is what turns a good and competent doctor into a healer. He is not talking about something superstitious but rather about the ability some people have to imagine themselves into the other – to have a specific eye for the other in order to know what is necessary (Saul, 2001). Imagination assists the nurse to see the possibilities that exist for a client even in situations where the client cannot. According to Jackson and McKergow (2002) there can be no progress without possibilities 'a future without possibility is a future without hope (Jackson and McKergow, 2002, p. 71). To see the possibilities we need imagination.

Imagination has other uses as well. Imagination is necessary when using the techniques of SFN such as the miracle question. In using the miracle question we are asking the client to see what might be and also to see the elements of a brighter future already existing in the present. It is a key to creativity and creativity is a key to helping people find or re find novel solutions to their problems.

Collaborative Puzzles

As has been discussed, solution focused nursing is relationship driven and the process of working in a solution focused way is as important as the outcomes – sometimes more so. The process of working with people can be therapeutic as much as the product. There will be many times when the techniques used in Solution-Focused Nursing do not yield the results we expect. However, it is never pointless even if we don't always get the results we would like. In working in solutions focused ways we are by our actions giving clients the message that they are unique individuals who have strengths and are capable of improving their situation (Hagan and Mitchell, 2001). Working with the client in collaborative ways using imagination and creativity we are also doing more than finding solutions, we are building a new way of working with people and a new way of viewing problems – seeing them as 'puzzles'. Viewing the problem as a puzzle takes away the blame focus and the focus on the past. In traditional ways of dealing with problems the cause of the problem or who or what is to blame, is often the focus. In working in solution focused ways in nursing, more time is spent on helping clients develop a clear vision for how they want the future to be. The past is helpful in identifying things that have worked before but this is refocused on how this knowledge can be used to reach a present or future goal (Webster, 1990). Seeing problems as puzzles helps clients and nurses work in a more creative and positive way. Puzzles have a different focus to problems and require people to think in a different way. Puzzles are shared. We seldom ask 'whose puzzle is it anyway?' We seldom say 'that's your puzzle' and of course we are unlikely to say 'who caused the puzzle in the first place?' Seeing problems as puzzles uses our imagination to reframe something old into something new. A problem becomes a puzzle. Unlike problems, puzzles imply solutions. Puzzles usually take creativity and a different way of looking at things to solve. Puzzles are often solved with the help of others and once you have solved one puzzle other puzzles will often be easier to solve.

Reader Activity: This activity is based around the miracle question. Ask yourself the following questions and write down your answers.

1. If a miracle occurred tonight and I woke up and I was a better nurse and worked in a more solution focused way what would be different?
2. What would clients and staff observe that would indicate there had been a change in my behaviour and ways of working with clients?

Reflecting on the answers that you have given to these questions, are any of the things you have listed happening now, even a little? List these and answer the following question.

3. What strategies could I use to ensure that I do more of these things in the future?

Having completed the exercise thus far you should have a list of things that you can do to improve your interactions with clients and work in a more solution focused way. There may be other things you can think of that do not appear on the list that you could also try. Add these to the list. We hope you feel keen to try these things out when next you are working with clients. However, we often start out with good intentions to try out new ways of working and improving on old ways but then we gradually fall back on old habits. So to help guard against this tendency, we would like you to open your diary and find the date three months from today's date. On that page write the answers to question 3. In three months time reflect upon the extent to which you have achieved your goal.

The Importance of Building Self-Esteem and Self-Efficacy

Nursing in a solution focused way helps people working thorough mental health transitions feel listened to and their experience valued. It helps clients see themselves as unique and with the capability and strengths to improve their lot (Hagen and Mitchell, 2001). The client is seen as experts in their own lives (Webster, Vaughn and Martinez, 1994). In more traditional ways of working with people there is often a tendency for the nurse to put him/herself in the role of problem solver. This puts undue pressure on the nurse to find solutions for, rather than with, the client. It also puts the client in a passive rather than active position in the relationship. Such passivity is unlikely to lead to future growth and the development of self-esteem and self-efficacy. By contrast, working in a solution focused way acknowledges the client as an expert in their own life and places the nurse in the position of ally and supporter. In this context the nurse can ask thoughtful solution focused questions of the client who may learn to value their own solution focused answers in turn building self-esteem and self-efficacy (the belief that I have the skills and power to do something about my own situation). This facilitative way of working utilizes the principles of:

- I know what I believe when I hear myself talk, and
- People are more likely to integrate and accept that which is reached by their own reasoning powers (Miller, 1983).

For example, in the case of Dave and Peter, when Peter reported that he is feeling much better and Dave replied, 'That's great! How did you do that?' This simple reply acknowledges that the improvement was the result of Peter's actions, not the qualities of Dave as expert nurse. Peter and Dave could then work together to develop other solutions. In developing strategies together Peter is using his own reasoning powers and is therefore more likely to accept the idea as a possible solution. This is far more powerful than the nurse offering a solution 'I think you should do'.

The story of Peter and Dave is left with them continuing to work together with Peter's mental health transitions as they arise as they inevitably do but in the process they are working together to find solutions and build Peter's capacity to cope with these transitions though the development of self-esteem and self-efficacy.

What are Mental Health Transitions?

Mental health transitions are times in our lives where transitions challenge our mental health. Two key points about transitions need emphasis. First, transitions are transient. Mental health transitions, like any other transition are not permanent. Of course this may not be obvious to the people who are undergoing these transitions. It is worth remembering that, for the most part, people with mental health issues will recover or at least improve. Even people with severe and enduring mental illness (such as Peter in the story) will have times when their mental health is in transition towards wellness. This is important and will help nurses and clients keep their present circumstances in perspective. It is also useful to remember this when looking for solutions or partial solutions to mental health puzzles. Nothing happens all the time and this being the case it is possible for the nurse to help the client look for exceptions. Exceptions are times when the problem is not there. Webster (1990) suggests a question to explore exceptions is: 'What is it that is going on when the problem is not there?' Exceptions offer a glimpse at some possible solutions and strengths already in use but often overlooked because of the client's and the nurse's tendency to focus on the problem.

Second, transitions move us to a different space and are seen in the context of the whole life of the individual. Problem focused ways of working with clients focus on negative aspects of the client's experience. From a solution focused nursing perspective the nurse and client focus on exceptions – times when the problem was not present – with a view to identifying strengths and solutions. This can have the effect of reframing the mental health to something more positive, something which has hidden within it the possibility of positive growth. This is not to romanticize or trivialize mental health transitions but rather to put them into the perspective of the person's overall life experience and by doing so help the person transit from them in a more positive and life affirming way.

Some Guiding Principles For SFN With Transitions In Mental Health

Building Engagement

Practice the techniques of Solution-Focused Nursing but remember that techniques used in the context of a strong therapeutic alliance will be more likely to be successful.

Being Creative

Use your and the client's imagination to see future possibilities and develop novel client centred solutions to get there.

Building Client Self-Esteem and Self-efficacy

The client is unlikely to find solutions and put them into practice unless in the process of doing so she or he is able to feel good about themselves and positive about their ability to change their circumstances.

Puzzles Not Problems

Working collaboratively on a puzzle to be solved is likely to yield more in the way of creative solutions than focusing on a problem.

Working Together with a Client is Never Pointless

Even if the techniques and solutions don't yield the results we expect, the way we work with the client can have a positive effect.

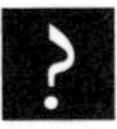

Group Activity: Part 1. With a small group of your colleagues, take a moment to reflect as a group upon your work as nurses. Remember the times with clients that you really felt that you made a connection, helped a client develop their strengths and assisted them to find solutions to cope with their current and future mental health transitions. Together list these under the heading 'Claims'.
For example. 'I claim that I assisted a client to develop strategies to deal with depression'.
Part 2. Next the group should discuss and list their concerns about working as nurses under the heading 'Concerns'.
For example 'I get anxious when working with people who exhibit aggression'.
Part 3. Once the group has listed their concerns, the group could return to the list of 'claims'. As a group discuss what is it that you did when working with clients that contributed to the 'claims' you identified? List these ways of working.
Part 4. Now return to your list of 'Concerns'. As a group discuss the ways of working that you identified in Part 4 and the extent to which you would be able to use these ways of working to assist you in overcoming your concerns.

Suggestions for Further Reading

Hagan, B., and Mitchell, D. (2001). Might within madness: Solution-focused therapy and thought-disordered clients. *Archives of Psychiatric Nursing, 15*(2): 86–93.

Lipchik, E. (2002). *Beyond technique in solution focused therapy: Working with emotions and the therapeutic relationship*. New York: Guilford Press.

Teacher notes to accompany this chapter can be found at www.palgrave.com/nursinghealth/mcallister

References

Hagan, B., and Mitchell, D. (2001). Might within madness: Solution-focused therapy and thought-disordered clients. *Archives of Psychiatric Nursing, 15*(2): 86–93.

Jackson, P., and McKergow, M. (2002). *The solution focus: What works at work*. London: Brealey.

Lewis, T., and Osborn, C. (2004). *Solution focused counseling and motivational interviewing: A consideration of confluence. Journal of Counseling and Development, 82*: 38–48.

Lipchik, E. (2002). *Beyond technique in solution focused therapy: Working with emotions and the therapeutic relationship.* New York: Guilford Press.

Miller, W. (1983). Motivational interviewing with problem drinkers, *Behavioural Psychotherapy, 11*(2), 147–172.

Miller, W., and Rollnick, S., (2002). *Motivational interviewing: Preparing people for change.* New York: Guilford Press.

Quick, E. (1996). *Doing what works in brief therapy: A strategic solution focused approach.* San Diego: Academic Press.

Saul, R. J. (2001). *On equilibrium.* Penguin Books, Toronto.

Walsh, K. (1999). Shared humanity and the psychiatric nurse-patient encounter. *The Australian and New Zealand Journal of Mental Health Nursing. 8*(1):2–9.

Walsh, K., McAllister, M., Morgan, A. and Thornhill, J. (2004). Motivating change: Using motivational interviewing in practice development. *Practice Development in Health Care*, 3(2): 92–100.

Webster, D. (1990). Solution-focused approaches in psychiatric/mental health nursing. *Perspectives in Psychiatric Care, 26*(4): 17–21.

Webster, D., Vaughn, K., and Martinez, R. (1994). Introducing Solution Focused Approaches to staff in Inpatient Psychiatric Settings. *Archives of Psychiatric Nursing 8*(4): 254–261.

CHAPTER 10

Solution-Focused Nursing with Survivors of Sexual Violence: A Cultural Context

Mary de Chesnay

Overview

This chapter will be an exploration of solution-focused nursing from a cultural context with special attention to working with survivors of domestic violence, incest and rape. One does not need to be working in remote villages to understand cultural differences and to appreciate the need for culturally competent skills. Cultural competence as a construct for nursing practice is fairly new in our language, but powerful as a goal in the continuous improvement of how we relate to clients and to each other as nurses. Nurses share a common culture of nursing even though we might come from many different countries or ethnic regions. Solution-focused, culturally competent nursing care represents a universal phenomenon that binds us as health care providers with a mission not only to cure disease, but also to promote healthy patterns and attributes in the people we serve. Rather than overlook differences by assuming that people's needs and desires are the same, this chapter will show how to talk with clients so that their cultural and sub-cultural identities are revealed and respected and how to work across cultural differences so that clients are more likely to be actively engaged in the health care encounter. There are many solutions that might be appropriate in any given situation, but some will not be congruent with the client's cultural values, norms and lifeways (activities of daily living). The challenge for practitioners is to find ways to bring solution-focused nursing care in line with culture.

To this end, three cases are presented to illustrate commonalities and differences inherent in three types of violence: battering, incest and rape. Though fictitious, the stories are developed from the author's experience conducting psychotherapy with several hundred clients who have experienced these types of violence. The individuals represent different cultural backgrounds in order to discuss culturally competent nursing intervention within the context of solution-focused therapy. However, although the author practices psychotherapy, the intention in this chapter is to frame solution-focused therapy as a nursing intervention and the strategies described are appropriate for all nurses who work with survivors of sexual trauma. Readers are encouraged to think about these stories as a starting place for intervention, not as a complete protocol because in real life, many other factors would be evaluated for relevance to specific people.

For the purposes of this chapter, culture is defined broadly as shared values, norms, beliefs, and lifeways of a group of people bound by either geography or common experience. By this definition, there can be a culture of violence as well as the more traditional notion of culture as shared ethnicity and geographic home. Evidence that solution-focused therapy transcends cultures is found in the many sources about the therapy from nurses and other practitioners around the world (McAllister, 2003; Park, 1997). This chapter presents a few culturally diverse cases from the United States but readers are encouraged to apply the principles to their own cultures.

A Model of Problem-Solving Therapy

As a family therapist and applied anthropologist, the author works clinically from a theoretical framework she developed in the 1980's that represents an early version of solution-focused therapy in the sense of using creative change strategies to produce change in outcomes. Therefore, this chapter might seem somewhat confusing without a brief historical review of the author's model, first published a number of years ago, since the perspective of solution-focused therapy presented in this chapter evolved from a specific model of psychotherapy (de Chesnay, 1983a, b). The author's model is slightly different from (though consistent with) the current model of solution-focused therapy as described in this book. For an excellent overview of the current approach to solution-focused therapy, refer to earlier chapters in this book and McAllister (2003).

In the early days of brief therapy, the focus was on problem-solving (Haley, 1978; Watzlawick, Weakland, and Fisch, 1974) and, though the intent was to solve specific problems identified by the client, the outcomes were often unspecified or vague. Yet, this new focus on solvable problems instead of hopeless symptoms represented a giant step forward in the development of psychotherapy because therapists began to understand that clients are autonomous human beings. With understanding came the realization that therapists must abandon their roles as benevolent dictators of treatment and present themselves as consultants or coaches.

The contribution of the early brief therapy proponents was profound because the shift in thinking represented a paradigm shift not just in terms of the time-limited nature of brief therapy, but most importantly, in terms of new hopefulness about positive change – change that could occur because clients were now being taught how to assume control of their lives. Magically, once therapists focused on solvable problems with creative strategies to achieve solutions, clients began to see that they could become 'unstuck' from their previous destructive patterns of behaviour. Helplessness and despair gave way to hope and action toward change.

The author's model (de Chesnay, 1983b) was an attempt to link the brief therapy communication model (Watzlawick, Weakland and Fisch, 1974) with the nursing process, itself a problem-solving model. The nursing process conceptualization used by the author was published in the 1970's (Brodt, 1978) and has been viable for many years in forms that vary little. The model generally includes the following steps: assessment (culminating in nursing diagnosis or statement of the problem,) plan, implementation and evaluation. The author's focus was on the nature of stating the problem and the development of interventions designed to solve the problem as it is framed.

Although conceived as a problem-solving model there are three aspects that make the author's model appropriate to consider in the context of solution-focused nursing therapy and the model was first applied to non-psychiatric problems. First, the model emphasized the client's strengths and resources and broke down difficult and complex problems that cannot be solved to simpler problems that can be solved, enabling the client to experience a series of small successes fast. Second, the model emphasized creative change strategies that departed significantly from the kinds of previous interventions. Finally, there was an emphasis on the therapist's respectful approach to the client. This approach is personified by thinking of the therapist as a consultant, an expert who assists the client toward a goal, but who recognizes that the client is in control of his or her life. Thus, the two major concepts of the model are problem framing and change strategies.

Problem-Framing

There are two ways to frame the problem: as an individual problem belonging to the person or as a system problem, meaning that persons are seen as subsystems and the problem is therefore owned by the system (family) instead of the individual who exhibits symptoms. The classic way of looking at the world in psychiatry is that individuals are mentally ill. This position is a conceptualization that the person owns the problem (individual problem framing.) Classic diagnostic terminology is derived from individual problem-framing.

Later, psychiatric clinicians discovered the family. Viewing psychiatric symptoms of individuals as a family problem logically leads to system problem-framing. For example, systemic practitioners are less concerned about the nature and manifestation of schizophrenia than about the system of failed communication patterns in families in which a member carries the schizophrenic label. The redefinition or reframing of the problem opens up a new world of interventions because strategies no longer have to be geared just toward an individual but rather to the whole family, who can be helped to behave differently toward the schizophrenic and thus effect positive change in the schizophrenic's behaviour.

Another example of reframing that might be used by therapists is the notion that resistance is healthy. Therapists are taught to think of resistance by patients to change as negative and unhealthy (more precisely, that patients who resist doing what their therapists tell them to do are unhealthy). A different view of resistance was presented by Wade (1997) who contended that people who seek therapy often have been subjected to violence and that to resist violence is healthy. Consistent with solution-focused therapy, Wade argued that people have a pre-existing ability to resist violence and abuse and that the focus of therapy should be the person's response to the violence rather than how he or she was affected by the abuse.

Change Strategies

The traditional notion of change is that the burden of change is on the individual. For example, 'John needs to learn how to control his anxiety; therefore, we will administer psychotropic drugs to help him.' An alternate way of describing the phenomenon of change is that the burden of change shifts from a vulnerable individual (the identified patient) to several individuals who are presumably less vulnerable and who can share the burden of change. If parents and siblings or spouses can be taught to act differently toward the identified patient, it is expected that the identified patient will change in reaction to the family's new ways of behaving toward the identified patient. This shift can occur only when the family is taught to reframe the problem from 'John is sick' to 'Our family has a problem with John's behaviour.'

The types of possible change are categorized as first-order or second-order (Watzlawick, Weakland and Fisch, 1974.) These authors defined change in two ways: change occurring within the system (first order) or change of the system itself (second order). First-order solutions are logically drawn from individual problem framing. For example, a patient has a symptom so a medication is given to alleviate that symptom-take an aspirin for a headache. In many cases this strategy is successful. But what does one do if first order solutions do not work? Typically, we try many different first order solutions. If aspirin does not work, we try another brand or a higher dose but these solutions represent more of the same.

In contrast, second-order change strategies might be viewed as changing the system of failed solutions. In the headache example, two examples of second order solution are either to redefine the headache as a serious health problem and to seek diagnostic testing or to conclude that aspirin alone will not reduce it and that decreased activity might so the person decides to go to sleep in the hope that the headache will be gone upon awakening. Both strategies break the cycle of the system of failed solutions and refocus on a different type of solution.

In schizophrenia, administering anti-psychotic medication to the patient is a first order change strategy because the expectation is that the patient is sick and can be cured through medication or, at least that the symptoms of schizophrenia can be alleviated. In contrast, developing a family intervention to react to the schizophrenic's delusions is a second order strategy because the focus of change is on the family who is said to own the problem, not the identified patient.

Similarly, if a young child is having a temper tantrum in a public place, the tantrum tends to escalate in direct proportion to the amount of attention the child receives. Most parents of such children react to the tantrum either by shouting at the child to stop (giving the child enormous secondary gain in the form of their undivided attention) or by trying to ignore the tantrum in which case everyone around the parent gives the child attention, embarrassing the parent who then shouts louder at the child to stop. One second order change strategy that has been successful in this situation is to remove the child to a private place and encourage the child to continue the tantrum alone until she or he is finished. Once the pay-off of secondary gain is removed (the attention for the tantrum is the reward) the child loses interest in continuing.

Reader Activity: Categorize each of the following statements as either individual or system problem-framing.
'I know my husband loves me, but he has a real problem showing it'
'Our family has a problem communicating with each other'
'My supervisor hasn't figured out how to manage effectively'
'Our organization is not good about celebrating people's accomplishments'
'My professor writes bad exams'
'I would like my professor's help to learn why I did not do well on the exam'

The Model Applied to Violence

In practicing psychotherapy for many years, the author has successfully implemented problem framing and change techniques in her practice with survivors of violence. In point of fact, the term *survivor* is an excellent example of the new approach to psychotherapy. When therapists learned to refer to victims as survivors (reframing) they shifted from the problem-solving mode to the solution-focused mode. This deceptively simple step opened up a whole new way of thinking as the focus shifted from the problem to the solution. Keeping the focus on the problem and designing strategies around solving each sub-problem works well in clinical work. However, this kind of problem-solving approach tends to be a constant reminder to the survivor of the violent episode. The newer model of solution-focused therapy extends the therapy to reframe the negative experience into a positive reaction to the negative situation and healthy coping. That is, the therapy is designed to help the 'victim' see herself or himself as a survivor who can hopefully become stronger yet by placing the violent experience within a context that represents only a small part of life experience.

The Model within a Cultural Context

Violence is inherent in many cultures and violence against the vulnerable is particularly insidious to those of us who hold the value that a society should protect its weak and not allow members of the society to exploit them. The United States is a country of many cultures, a country with a rich diversity of human beings whose families or who themselves came from other countries with distinct yet sometimes conflicting cultural norms and values. There are many challenges associated with finding ways to respect diversity yet find common goals. The United States is not alone in being a heterogeneous society and, while the examples in this chapter are designed in the United States, readers from many other countries with similar richness in their citizenry can adapt these ideas for their own cultures. The important lesson here is to pay attention to culture-in all its richness.

To this end, the notion of problem framing and change strategies might be extended to cultural ways of looking at problems and solutions. For example, individual problem framing might be viewed as attempting to attribute behaviours to people because they are of certain races or ethnicities. Statements such as the following are examples of individual problem-framing:

'She allows herself to be abused because she is a good Muslim'
'She is a victim of incest because that happens a lot in Appalachia'
'She was raped because she went on a blind date and he turned out to be bad'.

It is important to distinguish that both individuals of the culture and outsiders might hold these beliefs, but the statements are still individual ways of looking at the problem-leading to ineffective (first order) solutions. There is implied blame against the 'victim' and the reader is left with the idea that things are hopeless.

In contrast, consider the following statements that exemplify system problem-framing:

'If she (a Muslim woman) left her abusive husband, she is likely to be shunned by her friends and family'.
'An Appalachian child who is sexually abused has few resources to turn to, given the isolation of her home'.
'Women who go on blind dates can be helped to develop protective strategies'.

In these scenarios, there are ways to develop change strategies that go beyond the individual woman's behaviour. For example in the case of the Muslim woman, one would want to help her to develop a support system within the Muslim community or, failing that, outside the community. Appalachian children still are covered by social services who might be taught to do better case-finding. Women should not have to avoid blind dates, but they might be helped to make certain self-protective contingency plans, such as using their own transportation until getting to know the man.

There is much to learn about culture, but one of the most important concepts to consider is one's own ethnocentric biases, the beliefs we hold that our own cultural ways are the right ones – or at least that we are familiar with our own cultural norms and values and so consider those of others to be less important. Ethnocentric bias is an important layer in the overall effectiveness of a nurse working with individuals who are not of the same cultural group.

Reader Activity: Take a moment to think of your own culture in whichever way you usually define yourself and your family. Do you define yourself culturally by religion, ethnicity or national origin-or some other way? Are you a member of a homogeneous society or would you say that your country is heterogeneous? What are the values, norms, and lifeways of your own culture?

Sandra's Story: Domestic Violence

Sandra is a 31 year old pregnant, white, rural Appalachian woman with 4 children and she was referred by a battered women's shelter for psychotherapy when she exhibited suicidal ideation in a group session at the shelter. She presented to the nurse-psychotherapist as somewhat depressed but denied that she was truly suicidal. Rather, she informed the nurse that her statements to the group were a cry for help: 'I just wanted someone to know how much pain I was in [when talking about her abusive husband]'.

During the intake interview, Sandra stated that she had told her husband she was pregnant and that he beat her, while berating her for becoming pregnant. 'Although he beat me before, it was never like this. I didn't want to get pregnant again, but he won't use protection-or let me-and it just happened.' She indicated that in the past when her husband beat her, he would then want sex and would claim to love her so she forgave him and endured her life.

She related the story of how she had run away – first taking her children to her sister's home in another state, because she did not want to lose her baby. However, her sister did not have enough room and she was not able to stay long. When she left her sister's home, Sandra and her children had no funds to return home so they remained in the city and slept on the street. Sandra lived in fear that her husband would find her and that if she returned to him, the beatings would only worsen.

Reader Activity: Write down three beliefs you have about why men batter.

The Cultural Context

That Sandra lived in rural Appalachia of the United States is important to know in order to provide a cultural context of her as white, of Scottish-Irish descent and poor. Her story could be told by many women around the world who live in isolated regions with similar cultural values. In Appalachia, a mountainous, fairly isolated region of the United States that extends along the eastern seaboard, women are expected to provide emotional strength to their families and to be the primary caretakers. They are expected to place their families' needs above their own and because they are poor and isolated, they are at risk for injury and violence (Patton, 2005). Appalachian children are at risk from family violence and sexual abuse (Costello *et al.*, 1997). Given the isolation and poverty of Appalachian women in general, Sandra's story might be considered typical, though, of course, not all Appalachian men batter their wives and children.

Intervention

It is tempting to blame Sandra's husband for being abusive and to do so would be an example of individual problem-framing. However, individual problem framing leads to first order change strategies, such as providing an anger management program for the husband, which would be hard to implement in this situation. Assigning responsibility or ownership of the problem to the husband is ineffective because he is not available to change nor is evidence available that he might wish to change. To recruit him into the therapeutic session would be to place Sandra at further risk.

Similarly, it is possible to frame the problem as Sandra's problem of allowing herself to be abused, but this is not helpful and might be construed as insulting since she actually has taken action against being abused by leaving home with her children. Again, this would be individual problem framing leading to first order change strategies, or change within Sandra in terms of her attitudes and choices.

Framing the problem in such a way that it can be solved and that the principles of solution-focused nursing are applied in this case would involve working with Sandra to identify strengths and resources that she might use to better her situation. Doing so would be an example of system problem-framing, since the therapist would recognize that there is a culture of violence and that Sandra and her husband are caught up in a cycle that they could not break until Sandra left home. The strategies for intervention shift from Sandra's behaviour to her strengths and resources. A culturally competent care plan for Sandra might include the following strategies and solutions.

Some strategies might be:

1. Get her to acknowledge her courageous decision to leave home. A typical individual problem framing and highly negative response to women who are battered is 'Why didn't you leave him earlier?' Focusing on her courage at leaving him at all is much more beneficial.
2. Help her to reframe her husband's behaviour as his problem, not her fault. The powerful norm Appalachian women have to support their families makes it easy for them to feel guilty and internalize the blame for abuse.
3. Assist her to find prenatal care while expressing respect for her decision to keep the baby.
4. Help her identify shelters and social services agencies that might assist her for short-term housing while expressing confidence in her problem-solving abilities.
5. Help her to break down the many problems associated with daily living into small manageable goals that she can solve quickly and experience small successes.

The solutions the nurse expects are:

1. Sandra reframes her leaving as a sign of courage, not weakness.
2. Sandra reframes her abuse as her husband's issue, not hers.
3. Sandra states she feels supported in her decision to keep the child. (Alternatively, Sandra has an opportunity to consider other options related to her pregnancy with a non-judgmental listener-the nurse.)
4. Sandra finds temporary housing that is safe for herself and her children.
5. Sandra solves other problems of daily living while developing a long-term plan for job, housing, etc and expresses that she feels successful at coping.

Reader Activity: What other strategies and solutions might you consider?

Zena's Story: Incest

Zena is a 9 year old African American girl who was admitted to the inpatient psychiatric unit by her mother when her father was prosecuted for incest. The mother contends that Zena is 'mentally ill' and that she 'made up the story' of her father's abuse. Zena's story is that her unemployed father first came into her room at night two years earlier when she was 7 years old. At the time, her mother had taken a job as supervisor on the night shift at a factory. Zena said that her father explained that her mother was gone too much and that he and

Zena needed to comfort each other. 'Comfort' first meant holding and touching, but after a few nights he progressed to sexual intercourse. Zena indicated she tried to resist because 'it hurt' but he would not stop. Furthermore, he told her that they had a 'special relationship' and that her mother would be terribly jealous if she learned about their closeness. He indicated he would kill her if she told anyone, especially her mother. One morning while doing laundry, Zena's mother discovered blood on her underwear and asked her if she hurt herself. Zena told her about the abuse, but her mother's response was to accuse Zena of lying and she instructed Zena never to talk about this again. However, Zena disclosed to her school nurse when the nurse performed an exam for acute stomach ache. The school nurse referred Zena to social services, and the family was investigated. Although the father had been arrested, the mother and Zena were referred to a nurse-therapist.

Reader Activity: Under what conditions would you want to believe the mother rather than Zena in this story? Take a moment to write down your thoughts, including your first reaction to the story.

The Cultural Context

There are two cultures represented in this story: an ethnic culture (African American) and the culture of poverty. That Zena's mother worked and her father did not meant that, although Zena's mother is the breadwinner, there is a powerful force at work between the parents in which the mother protects the father's masculinity by deferring to him and believing him over her own child. In the United States, there is systematic racism regarding African Americans that is no less insidious since desegregation. In some ways, African American women have been able to achieve more than African American men, since they are perceived as less threatening by the dominant majority-white men. Therefore, from a cultural point of view, it is not surprising that Zena's mother would try to protect her husband first.

The mother's choice of action is hard to understand for people who view the child's needs as taking precedence over the father's. The ethnocentric bias of the dominant majority would be that children should be protected at all costs and that the child's needs come first. However, this is a moral position and may not be relevant to Zena's mother. Unfortunately, the father in this story would be perceived as typical and there could be a backlash against other African American men who do not abuse their children. This is racism excused on the basis of placing the child's needs first. The mother needs to be approached delicately, not in a blaming manner, because she is caught between a rock and hard place – to believe and protect her husband or her child. In a sense she is successful in her attempt to protect her family – the trick is to get her to learn the difference between supporting her husband and accepting bad behaviour. In addition, the mother needs to find a way to protect her daughter – the first step might be to believe her.

Intervention

For Zena and her mother, the problem needs to be reframed form 'Zena is lying' to 'Zena is telling the truth' about what happened to her. Furthermore, it is critical that the mother be supported for trying to be a 'good wife' while at the same time helping her to see the truth in Zena's story. Accusing the mother of being a co-abuser is destructive not only to the family, but also to the nursing care and would be classic individual problem framing with only one solution-to remove the child from the home.

Some strategies might be:

1. Get the mother to acknowledge Zena's story and to express respect for Zena's courage at coming forward.
2. Help the mother to reframe her husband's behaviour in such a way that she recognizes he did something wrong while simultaneously expressing empathy for her supporting him.
3. Assist Zena to understand that she did the right thing by coming forward.
4. Help Zena's mother to develop a plan for life without her husband, at least temporarily, and to decide what to do when he is released from prison.
5. Help Zena to understand that the abuse was not her fault and that she is not alone.

The solutions the nurse expects are:

1. Zena's mother reframes Zena's story from a lie to the truth and expresses regret for not believing her.
2. Zena's mother reframes her husband's behaviour from acceptable to not acceptable and acknowledges the need to hold him accountable.
3. Zena acknowledges that she understands it was wrong of her father to abuse her and wrong of him to threaten her and that she was right to come forward.
4. Zena's mother identifies resources to help her protect Zena in the future. (One example is child care-previously, the husband 'took care of Zena' while the mother worked.)
5. Zena expresses that she understands that she is not to blame.

Reader Activity: What other strategies and solutions might you consider?

Martin's and Sue's Story: Rape

Martin and Sue are an unmarried, affluent white couple in their late 20's who seek therapy after Sue was raped by a stranger while taking the bus home from work one night. She reported the rape but the man has not been found. The couple had planned to marry, but Sue postponed the wedding because as she states, 'I can't stand to be touched.' The couple live in a luxury apartment in a large city and Sue works in an area of town that is considered safe by day but dangerous by night. Martin and Sue are both professionals and have high-paying jobs. They are focused on building their careers and spend their free time having dinner parties with their circle of like-minded friends. Prior to the rape, they attended the symphony, theater and ballet and were active in local charities, but Sue has become withdrawn and does not like to leave their apartment except for work. They have stopped socializing with their friends because Sue is 'embarrassed'. She now takes the taxi to work, but the couple live beyond their means and taxis are expensive. They seek help because Sue is aware that their lives have changed dramatically, yet she cannot seem to find a way past the rape. During the first session in which Sue tells the therapist about the rape, she explains that she does not think she 'will ever get over it.' She is considering ending the engagement because she is not sure she can ever have sex again and she frames herself as to blame, indicating she loves Martin: 'It's my fault and it is not right for him to have to deal with me. He deserves better.' Martin insists that he loves Sue and is willing to wait for her to get past the rape. In fact, he seems to constantly reassure her – an activity with good intentions which backfires because the more he reassures her, the harder she finds it to believe him.

Reader Activity: Write down your reaction to the following statement: 'Well, if she was foolish enough to be walking alone at night in a city, she was asking for it'.

The Cultural Context

Culture is not just about race, ethnicity and poverty. Martin and Sue are affluent white professionals and their cultural norms, values and lifeways are important to them. Being raped has torn Sue's comfortable world apart and significantly affected her fiancé as well. The idea that Sue's sexual life must be over is not uncommon for rape survivors, but it is possible to work with this couple to revive their relationship. For many women, being raped is such a violent and frightening event that they only want to forget about it, but in trying hard to forget, they are instead focusing on the rape (don't think of a pink elephant). The harder they try not to think of the rape, the more they do until they are paralysed. This is a classic first order change strategy.

Some therapists work with survivors on this focusing behaviour as a way of helping them to see the event in context, but this is a first order change strategy that may backfire. Instead with women who are reacting this way, I like to spend much time in therapy talking about everything but the rape before we talk about the rape, as a way of helping the woman to see herself as successful in life and healthy (she survived, didn't she? So whatever she did was the right thing to do).

It might also be good to enlist Martin as a co-therapist. Guiding him in how he might respond to her in the best way might be the most therapeutic way of working with Sue. It would be important to help Martin reframe his response to Sue from 'How do we get our sex life back?' to 'How can we develop our relationship in other areas while we're waiting for this experience to settle?' All interventions should be framed with confidence that Sue can get past the experience-it just takes some people longer. Martin's constant reassurance, given with the best intentions, has the unfortunate effect of reminding Sue daily that she was raped, thereby paradoxically reinforcing the trauma for her. Martin's anxiety is communicated to her and represents a continuous form of pressure on Sue, thereby creating a paradoxical effect – the opposite of the intended effect. The closer he comes, the more she backs away-a classic first order change strategy. He needs to back away and enable her to come to him (a second order change strategy) but this is extremely hard to do. Sometimes first order strategies seem to be the most natural, and it is difficult to think of alternates when one is highly anxious. So Martin tries even harder and the harder he tries, the more he fails to achieve his goal of reassuring Sue and the vicious cycle continues.

Intervention

Some strategies might be:

1. Assist Sue to frame the rape experience as only one event in her life. To do so may involve expressing her anger, sadness, fears and anxieties.
2. Discuss with Sue her many areas of control, self-confidence and successes in life.
3. Enlist Martin as a co-therapist and work with him on ways to relieve the guilt and pressure Sue feels over the change in her reaction to him.
4. Help the couple come up with specific new things to do together so that their bond continues to grow without the pressure of sex. This often leads to a renewal of their sexual life because the pressure is off and they are not focused on sex. For example, they have never attended a baseball game together and, while neither particularly enjoys baseball, attending a game enables them to share a novel experience. They may never attend another game, but they might decide it is something new for them to do together, thereby creating another reframe of how they can spend time together.

The solutions the nurse expects are:

1. Sue's feelings of guilt, anger and fear dissipate as she gradually places the rape within the context of her life.
2. Sue focuses on a new aspect of her life that she wants to bring back into focus such as a new goal at work.
3. Martin shifts from constantly reassuring Sue that he still loves her to backing off and giving her the space to enable her to feel control over her life and body again while simultaneously being emotionally available to her.
4. The couple spend more time doing fun things together. Paradoxically, it is during such relaxing times when they are truly just having fun with each other that the desire for sexual intimacy returns.

Reader Activity: What other strategies and solutions might you consider?

Solutions

In all three stories of sexual violence, the interventions are designed to emphasize the solutions rather than the original problems of abuse. Readers may not like the interventions given. That is perfectly fine because there are many solutions to every problem – the challenge is to develop a varied menu of potential solutions. Thinking about systems instead of individuals helps the therapist be creative in working with clients on possible solutions. If one solution fails, then learn to fail successfully – by moving on to another solution. This idea of learning to fail successfully applies to the nurse as well as the client.

Solutions should be framed in such a way that the client can experience a series of small successes rather than setting goals that are intimidating in scope. For example, in Sandra's case, she needs to have a plan for how she will live and support her children if she does not return to her husband. Zena's mother needs to be helped to focus on her child's needs. Sue and Martin need to experience a new level of intimacy so that they can reframe sex as only one aspect of their love for each other.

All these solutions are examples of second order change strategies and all involve reframing the original violent problem in profound ways. The reframed problems, issues or goals are not just owned by the client. The therapist must understand how to reframe as well. For example, it does absolutely no good to shift the blame to someone else while trying to get the client to stop blaming herself.

In Sandra's story, it might be tempting to spend time in therapy talking about how bad her husband is, but that will not help Sandra to figure out how to support her children. The solution focus for Sandra needs to be consistent with her culture in emphasizing how strong she is and how much she loves her children.

For Zena and her mother, the shift is from blaming the victim (Zena) to protecting her. Holding the father accountable might be construed as blaming him, and in a sense, one can argue that he should be blamed, but blaming and holding accountable are not the same thing. It is not cost-effective to spend valuable therapy time dwelling on the father's failings which would only keep the focus on him and off the child. For Sue and Martin, reframing love as including more than sex is a healthy solution. Blaming herself is not a solution but blaming the rapist, while morally justified, is also not practical because then the attention is on the rapist and the event instead of on Sue's future.

Conclusion

The literature on solution-focused nursing is evolving and much attention is being given to the topic in the nursing, medical and counselling disciplines. This chapter has been an attempt to find a frame of reference that incorporates the best elements of finding solutions to problems of sexual violence. There are many ways to look at the stories presented here and many effective ways of working with people in similar situations. The crucial lessons are to frame the problem in such a way that it can be solved, to develop creative change strategies that make use of the client's strengths, to focus on small solutions to enable the client to feel successful early in therapy and to consider culture (your own and the client's) as a major variable in care.

References

Brodt, D. (1978). The nursing process. In N. Chaska (ed.) *The nursing profession: Views through the mist.* New York: McGraw-Hill.

Costello, E.J., Farmer, E., Angold, A., Burns, B., and Erkanli, A. (1997). Psychiatric disorders among American Indian and white children in Appalachia: The Great Smoky Mountains Study. *American Journal of Public Health, 87*(5), 827–832.

de Chesnay, M. (1983a). The creation and dissolution of paradoxes in nursing practice. *Topics in Clinical Nursing, 5*, 73–80.

de Chesnay, M. (1983b). Problem-solving in nursing. *Image: The Journal of Nursing Scholarship, 15*(1), 8–11.

Haley, J. (1978). *Problem-solving therapy.* San Francisco: Jossey-Bass.

McAllister, M. (2003). Doing practice differently: Solution-focused nursing. *Journal of Advanced Nursing, 41*(6), 528–535.

Park, E. (1997). An application of brief therapy to medicine. *Contemporary Family Therapy: An International Journal, 19*(1), 81–90.

Patton, C. (2005). Rural Appalachian women: A vulnerable population. In M. de Chesnay (ed), *Caring for the vulnerable* (pp. 277–282). Sudbury, MA: Jones and Bartlett.

Wade, A. (1997). Small acts of living: Everyday resistance to violence and other forms of oppression. *Contemporary Family Therapy, 19*(1), 23–39.
Watzlawick, P. Weakland, J. and Fisch, R. (1974). *Change*. New York: W.W. Norton.

Answers to the First Reader Activity: Categorize each of the following statements as either individual or system problem-framing.

'I know my husband loves me, but he has a real problem showing it.' (Individual)

'Our family has a problem communicating with each other.' (System)

'My supervisor hasn't figured out how to manage effectively.' (Individual)

'Our organization is not good about celebrating people's accomplishments.' (System)

'My professor writes bad exams.' (Individual)

'I would like my professor's help to learn why I did not do well on the exam.' (System)

CHAPTER 11

Living with Chronic Illness

Glenn Gardner and Anne Gardner

Overview

This chapter is about care for patients in hospital who have co-morbid chronic illnesses. As previously discussed, hospital nursing has traditionally been focused upon a concerted, therapeutic attention to an acute illness or injury. For example when patients enter hospital for surgery the nursing focus is on preparing them for the operation, attending to their needs and well-being during surgery, assisting their recovery from anaesthetic, supporting pain relief and healing, and coaching and assisting their return to previous levels of function post operatively. Similarly, the patient admitted for an acute medical illness is reliant upon nursing care that delivers interventions relevant to the health condition, monitors the patient's response to these interventions, provides symptom relief for manifestations of their illness and supports their emotional and biophysical requirements daily during the admission. You will find that nursing still does involve these activities but the patient outcomes you are working towards are different from this one dimensional, curative focus. Over the past decade the demographic of the acute hospital patient has changed. Patients who are admitted to hospital for an acute illness or injury are increasingly likely to have at least one existing chronic illness in addition to their acute

Reader Activity: Chronicity can mean many things: Create a table that lists chronic health conditions and suggest potential biological, psychological and social problems that may require amelioration and adaptation.

Chronic Condition	Biological	Psychological	Social
Multiple Sclerosis	Pain	Anxiety re role loss	Isolation from reduced mobility

health concern and the nursing care you practice in the hospital setting will include chronic disease management.

Before we begin it is helpful for readers to reflect on existing knowledge about the topic and to draw upon insights already gained in the reading of this book.

The Experience of Chronic Care in Hospitals

The literature tells us that inpatients in acute care hospitals globally, are increasingly elderly (Sager and Rudberg, 1998), are highly likely to suffer multiple chronic diseases (Redelmeier *et al.*, 1998) and have shorter hospital stays for treatment of their acute illness (Hogstel and Cox, 1995). It is clear that the presence of ongoing underlying chronic medical conditions, in combination with a decline in regenerative ability and a curtailed hospital-based recovery time, are significant factors affecting acute health care outcomes for the elderly. Much of the literature on various aspects of acute hospital care of the elderly highlights the complex and problematical nature of that care.

For many people the experience of chronic illness is about being in-between health and illness. Sometimes they experience intermittent acute illnesses or acute exacerbation of a chronic condition, and recover but remain unwell and unable to return to work and full-time responsibilities. The person living with a chronic condition can find themselves in a liminal state, feeling as though they belong nowhere and not having the skills to cope with this in-between place. Understanding this concept of liminality (van Gennep, 1960) may help nurses to more clearly see that their role is to facilitate movement across this threshold (Buchanan, 1997).

Reader Activity: Recall the major transitions that you and your family have so far experienced.
Sometimes these transitions are marked with ritual and also ritually remembered: birthdays and anniversaries, for example.
What transitions in health are usually marked in these ways?
How might transitions in the experience of chronic care be marked or enriched?

Learning to live with on-going problems or to adapt to a changed way of living are some of the challenges for people with chronic illness. Nurses have a role in helping people to de-centre problems, to reveal and enhance hidden sources of strength, resilience and social connections. Working in this context, nurses utilize goal directed strategies to move towards recovery and adaptation. Nurses working with clients who have chronic illnesses do not need to place the problem at the centre of the nurse–client interaction. As this chapter shows, it is possible to foreground the presence of both problems and strengths even in the midst of complex and enduring ill-health. Working in this context requires creativity, problem-solving and solution searching to maximize potentials by building on strengths, achievements and capacity.

Comorbidity management in partnership with the patient is now a central aspect of acute care nursing. The hospital admission is for the patient an interruption, and complication to their ongoing self management of chronic illness. We recently conducted a study to examine the health care of patients in the acute hospital who also have comorbid chronic illness (Gardner and Osborne, 2005). For most of the participants in the study the health management was characterized by a disease model, an approach to care that had the effect of overlooking the potential that a wellness model would offer. This was particularly relevant to the complex issues related to going home from hospital.

Learning to Live With Rather than Die from Disease

Several writers in the field of chronic illness stress the importance of a wellness model in learning to self manage chronic disease (Nolan and Nolan 1999, Verbrugge and Jette, 1994). An admission to hospital provides an important opportunity for nurses to work with patients to achieve long term solutions in living with chronic illness. In the following section we have supplied two stories in the words of the patients and their nurses. These stories will assist you to develop strategies for solution focused care.

Beryl's Story

Clinical summary: Beryl, is 83. She lives independently in her own home with her family. On admission she is alert, continent, self-caring and is independently mobile with a walking stick. She presented to Emergency with slurred speech, unsteady gait and was admitted as a general medical patient with a differential diagnosis of Cerebral Vascular Accident (CVA) or Transient Ischaemic Attack (TIA) for investigation. She has several pre-existing chronic illnesses: polymyalgia, atrial fibrillation, vascular disease, angina, chronic obstructive respiratory disease (CORD) and gastroesophageal reflux.

Of course, Beryl would tell her story quite differently. Take a closer look at how she described her experience.

> I have two illnesses in my life – pneumonia and shingles that's all I've had. Oh I had polymyalgia which is um, inflammation of muscles, I had that. Oh and Angina, Mm, it's very mild. I take cardizem and uh … . oh, Isordil. This has been going on I suppose for about, four or five years or so.
>
> I had an ultrasound it was yesterday, but they haven't changed anything. (when I had the pneumonia) It left me with a (clears throat) you know I have got to do that quite often. They think I'm choking on food here. I know, I know I'm not and my husband would know I'm not, I irritate him (laughter) he says have you got to do that? (Clears throat). The polymyalgia, it's the inflammation of the muscles. I was

> trying to make them do what I was doing at, about seventy I suppose. Ah what they couldn't do at seventeen.
>
> I was over, you know working too hard. But I got rid of it. Burns itself out, I was on prednisone about ten years but it burns itself out. The angina tablets haven't changed in hospital, except they changed the brand. They explained they didn't have the same brand as what I've been given by the specialist.
>
> The first couple of days I didn't have any control (over the situation). But ah, you know I can speak up now. I made sure I found out about (my illnesses) when I got them. I, you know I'm not a great one for taking tablets and I wanted to find out what I was taking and what I was taking them for.
>
> I do hope I can go home soon. I will be confident to continue with the angina. so long as I can write. I can't write like I used to you know but I'll conquer that.
>
> I have a GP, but the other fellow (the hospital specialist) he's sort of just watching me you know. Nothing is out of control. I made sure I found out about it (illnesses) when I got them.,You know I'm not a great one for taking tablets and I wanted to find out what I was taking and what I was taking them for.
>
> This stroke has got me worrying a bit you know, but, not as worried as getting home to my husband. He's, he's not really coping with all the looking after himself yet and I feel as though I don't walk well enough to get home. They are absolutely marvellous here. The attention is marvellous. [At this stage Beryl was crying and distressed, the interview was discontinued].

As this story shows there are many patients who are admitted to hospital for an acute illness or injury who also have an existing chronic illness. Beryl's situation is not unusual. She is a patient in hospital, she is sick and needing attention. In this narrative Beryl gives several cues that could direct her nursing care towards a solution focus.

Reader Activity: Analyse Beryl's narrative.
Identify the strengths that Beryl expresses in this narrative. How could you use these strengths to work with Beryl for her to achieve long term personal development within her chronic illness?

Beryl's story also raises the important notion of liminality. In nursing and health care, liminality refers to the experience of being in between. Literally, liminality is the word for the threshold moment, and comes from the Latin word meaning the centerline of the door way. Liminality is the moment of crossing over and marks a state of transition, where new becomes old, or sick becomes well. In cultural terms, there are many rituals to mark liminal stages and thus faciltiate safe passage through the transition, but in health care, many of these transitions are not safely facilitated, and so they constitute crises. The challenge for solution focused nurses is to be alert to all potential transition phases and develop skills in being with, and working with, clients to assist adaptation.

Now read the narrative from Beryl's nurse.

> Beryl has angina and polymyalgia. That is all I can remember really. I never asked her how she would um, manage those comorbidities at home. She didn't ask any questions about them. She directs her own care, taking pills. She was very good with her pills. She was very 'with it' so I imagine she would take her pills every day. I think she was her husband's carer.
>
> We were never faced with any problems with her angina and her other illnesses that sort of thing – just her main acute issue. So no extra new information was given to her. Her current illnesses didn't impact on the care that we were giving. Her main problems were with mobility so, we were just helping her to the toilet and sitting her up in a chair and she's gone to Rehab now. If she did start having angina then she probably would have had something looked at like stress tests. But because it didn't occur um … I guess we could keep everyone in here for a million years to sort out their problems, but yeah.

The nurse's perspective reflects some of the practices that are a feature of the acute care environment. First, there was an assumption that if there is no obvious problem, usually indicated through the presence of symptoms, there is no need for action. Other studies have also shown that nurses in acute care settings often underestimate the total number of comorbidities that patients with chronic illness live with. This may result in lack of acknowledgement of the comprehensive care needs of these patients (Williams, 2004).

Second, when it comes to complex care, nurses can end up caring more for the system's functioning than they do for the patient. The nurse's frustration revealed in the statement 'we could keep everyone in here for a million years to sort out their problems', shows a tension in holding a primary concern for patients' well being whilst also recognizing a mandate for nurses to control the ward environment and to maintain order and efficiency in this space. The consequence of this is an emotional and physical burden for nurses that is seldom acknowledged.

Reader Activity: Draw upon your learning from other chapters in this book and the activity you conducted above. Write your own "nurse's narrative" describing how you would bring a solution focus to Beryl's issues about **going home**.

Another story highlights different issues.

Dot's Story

Clinical summary: Dot is 69. She lives alone in a retirement unit. She is self-caring, continent and is independently mobile with a walking stick. She presented to Emergency with cellulitis causing ulceration of her large toe leading to decreased sensation possibly requiring amputation, and trans ischaemic attack/angina. She was admitted as a general medical patient. Her pre-existing illnesses included non-insulin dependent diabetes mellitus, previous myocardial infarct, mild diverticulitis, peripheral venous diabetic ulcers, retinopathy, and peripheral neuropathy.

Dot's own words give a deeper insight to her health situation.

> Well I have um diabetes and have had since 1983. I have lost a lot of blood flow in my extremities, mainly in the feet. ... and this is causing me problems with a sore on my foot. And it's something I've known that diabetics can have trouble with plus heart and apparently kidneys too. ... but so far I seem to have avoided the kidney problem (laughter). I have had high blood pressure since 1971, and I had a heart attack last July which is far as I know is related to the diabetes. But I don't always understand the details of the sickness I just try to pick up as much as I can about what I should and shouldn't do.
>
> I don't have any trouble at home, you know, as I've got older of course there is not as much house work to do. I can mange my own washing and ironing and general tidying up. My daughter's very good and if I need a hand she will do things for me, but generally speaking I do it myself. With the diabetes is it just tablets. Oh I take the blood sugar. I'm supposed to take it every day sometimes around 4 or 5 times a week I take it. I haven't talked to anyone about my BP or diabetes – they, have referred me to the dietician, but they've been more or less attending to the problem that I came in with.
>
> I've, gained a little bit of information about what they may have to do to me, like I may lose a toe yet. But um, I don't think I have learnt anything new.
>
> The trouble is, if something was there I'd read it, but I don't know whether, um, I could apply things to myself or not. But ah, I suppose it would be handy if there was information that there may be something that I'd pick up that would help me day to day.

In this narrative Dot frequently talks about her need for more knowledge and a better understanding of her conditions. One of the findings from our study into chronic illness in the acute environment was that nurses and patients both recognized the important role that information played in self and shared management of chronic and acute illness. However, there were different perspectives on the imperatives for knowledge. Nurses mostly operated from a professional expertise model whilst the patients often perceived themselves as holding their own expertise about their health problems and their information needs were related to relevance and personalized information needs.

Reader Activity: Draw up a list of the things that Dot is telling you she would like to know more about.

Draw up a list of the things that Dot has said that may reinforce her perception of her own wellness and *living with* her chronic diseases. What questions would you like to ask Dot to better identify her skills and capacity that you can both work on to improve her sense of self-efficacy, well being and self management.

Now read the narrative from Dot's nurse.

> Dot has cardiac problems, ischaemic heart disease, hypertension and sometimes she gets angina.
>
> The doctors think she's got some peripheral changes in her feet and that's resulted in an ulcer on her toe that hasn't healed. Like a lot of diabetics, she'd had to have her toes amputated, they weren't viable, she now has osteomyelitis. So there were some pretty harsh antibiotics as well as the toe amputation. She doesn't seem to realise how important it is, she just hasn't quite taken it in.
>
> I don't know how this is managed at home. Now we're looking at discharging her home in the next couple of days.
>
> So we need wound care at home, we need support with the medications, I think she has a supportive family, meals on wheels she'll need, we need to get her up and going, we need to get her mobile again so we got the physio in. We had a case meeting about her this morning. The physio, the dietician, the pharmacist, plus the medical team and the nursing team were there. All this would have been discussed.
>
> From my point of view I was happy that she rested for a while, with that foot.
>
> We haven't educated her at all about her diabetes and angina. I really think that she's happy to go along with whatever the doctor's say and if the doctor says you have to have the amputation she'll have it. ... not that there is anything wrong with any decision. But I think the thing to worry about is now she's lost one toe what can we do? She needs to ask 'what can I do to keep the rest of my toes'? I don't think she's asking the question.
>
> I don't think, we can fit in education. From the time angle, we are very busy – but also the patient is not ready to be educated yet.
>
> I think that her health status is poor I do honestly. If she was my mum I'd be ... (the nurse starts to cry), I'd be getting the whip out and going you know lets try a bit more. I'd be saying we need to keep those sugars under control, because it's such a serious thing. I don't think she's made the link between uncontrolled diabetes and her toe. I think she just thinks it's bad luck. I just mean it needs to be a comprehensive approach.

I think, if you listen carefully to what this nurse is saying you may recognize some of the values and imperatives that you have been learning as you work through the chapters in this book. The nurse is demonstrating many of the attributes that we value for excellent SFN care. She is patient-centred, empathetic, and technically competent. The important missing element in her strategy and vision for Dot's care is that her focus is on the *problem* related *to* Dot's health/illness rather than the *solution*. She is also working within the prevailing paradigm of care that is related to disease and disease management. This results in a simplification of Dot's complex health situation. The narrative indicates that the nurse can see the direction that she and Dot should take, but she lacks the solution focused nursing knowledge and skills to get them there.

Reader Activity:

- Analyse the nurse's narrative.
- List those statements/sentiments that resonate with your understanding of a solution-focused approach to nursing care.
- Re-order some of the situations she describes. For example who is missing from the case management meeting?

This story reveals what is a common tendency in health care that is dominated by a medico-scientific paradigm – nursing from a professional expertise model of patient teaching whilst the patients often perceive themselves as holding their own expertise about their health problems – a lay understanding. Two consequences for this tension become apparent: when patients draw upon their own theories to explain distressing symptoms they are not always brought to clinicians' attention because they are lay, rather than scientific understandings. Therefore, within this biomedical model of care, patient education is frequently scheduled, organized and delivered by the nurse with little attention to starting from and building on the patients' knowledge and expertise.

Despite Government initiatives over the past ten years to incorporate the patient in health management, the findings from our research indicate that health professionals and patients are not in accord with attitudes to information and teaching needs related to shared and self management of chronic disease. Notwithstanding their recognition of patients' own place in contributing to their care, the nurses mostly operated from a professional expertise model in that they determined where and what teaching would occur rather than engaging in dialogue about health information and management. Conversely the patients held their own theories and expertise related to their health concerns.

Solution-Focused Nursing

Nolan and Nolan (1999) suggest that most patients with chronic illness live with, rather than die from, their condition/s. Therefore rather than continue with the 'fight' against disease it is also important to assist people to develop personally within their illness. This approach is central to the values of nursing and holistic care. And yet the imperatives of nursing in the acute care environment determine that the structure of discharge planning centres around the acute condition, which as the above narratives illustrate, is at times in contradiction with the patients' need to 'live with' their conditions.

For many people, living with a chronic illness can be an experience of living in a liminal space – inbetween and belonging nowhere. The work of nursing with these patients is influenced by the culture of immediacy that is characteristic of the acute hospital environment and commonly results in a focus on the acute illness/episode and episodic, rather than coordinated, care of the patient's chronic diseases. It also tends to involve scant patient involvement in care outcomes and discharge planning. This was a limiting, and in some cases distressing, aspect of their work.

Tips for Working in Solution-Focused Ways with Clients Living with Chronic Illness (Remember the Joining Phase)

- Get to know the person and their chronic health conditions using a respectful approach.
- Try to frame any problems in a way that does not locate or lock it in as an individual problem belonging to the person. Remember that health is not merely the absence of disease, but a state of holistic well-being. Any problems need to be understood as located in the whole social system and this is also where solutions may be found.
- Try to identify the difficult and complex problems. Reframe any unhelpful labels into words that are more positive. 'Problems' can be 'challenges' or 'puzzles'.
- Then break them down into a series of simpler challenges that can be solved, enabling the person to experience a series of small successes fast.

Emphasize the Building Phase

- In situations where conditions continue and are not able to be cured, the building phase of SFN needs to emphasize adaptation and optimism.
- Emphasize the person's strengths and resources. He or she is living with a health care challenge and has found many ways to remain resilient.
- The client is unlikely to maintain motivation and hope unless she or he is able to feel good about themselves and positive about their ability to create changes.
- Be creative about change. Many of the strategies for change that you and the patient invent may depart significantly from more standard interventions. If they are safe, relevant and valued, then they will be important.
- Remember that working together with a client is never pointless. Even in situations where there are no technical or medical solutions, the human connection remains powerful. The way we work with clients can have a positive effect.

Move on to the Extending Phase

- Chronic conditions are by the nature ongoing, though your place in the person's life may wax and wane as acute issues arise, or when boosters of support or new puzzles emerge.
- Convey the attitude that the support you provide will be ongoing and that other supports and resources in the community exist.
- Together, work on accessing these resources and gathering up a strong web that nurtures, stimulates and challenges the client.

People with chronic health problems can learn to live with ongoing problems or to adapt to a changed way of living. Nurses have a hugely important role in helping people to decentre problems, to reveal and enhance hidden sources of strength, resilience and social connections. Our study showed that in-hospital management and discharge planning was dominated by the judgements and expertise of the health care staff, particularly the nurses. The patients' interviews frequently made reference to the nurses as a source of information and support and also demonstrated that the patients themselves held knowledge and expertise related to their chronic diseases. These factors together with patient determined outcomes must be taken into account in the selection or design of health-outcome assessment strategies and discharge planning. Working in this context, nurses can also utilize goal directed strategies to move towards recovery and adaptation.

This chapter has emphasized and reminded us that nurses working with clients who have chronic illnesses do not need to place the problem at the centre of the nurse–client interaction. It is possible to foreground the presence of both problems and strengths even in the midst of complex and enduring ill-health. Working in this context requires creativity, problem-solving and solution searching to maximize potentials by building on strengths, achievements, and capacity.

Group Activity: View the movie, *My left foot* (1989), which tells the story of Christy Brown who was born with cerebral palsy and overcame his severe disabilities to become a famous artist.

Work in teams to answer the following questions:

How do the characters' views of chronic illness differ?

If a nurse was introduced into this story, how might he or she facilitate safe passage through the family's transitions?

Suggestions for Further Reading

Bluebond-Langner, M. *(1996). In the shadow of Illness: Parents and siblings of the chronically ill child.* New Jersey, NJ: Princeton University Press.

References

Buchanan, T. (1997). Nursing our narratives: Towards a dynamic understanding of nurses in narrative tales. *Nursing Inquiry,4*, 80–87.

Gardner, G., and Osborne, S. (2005). *Investigating the care trajectory of elderly people with comorbidities in the acute care setting*. Report to Queensland Nursing Council. Brisbane.

Hogstel, M. O., and Cox, M. (1995). Hospital resources for care of acutely ill older persons. *Journal of Gerontological Nursing, 21*(11), 25–31.

Nolan, M., and Nolan, J. (1999). Rehabilitation, chronic illness and disability: the missing elements in nurse education. *Journal of Advanced Nursing, 29*(4), 958–966.

Redelmeier, D. A., Tan S. H., and Booth, G. L. (1998). The treatment of unrelated disorders in patients with chronic medical diseases. *The New England Journal of Medicine, 338*, 1516–1520.

Sager, M. A., and Rudberg, M. A. (1998). Functional decline associated with hospitalization for acute illness. *Clinics in Geriatric Medicine, 14*(4), 669–679.

Sheridan, J. (dir.). (1989). Video: *My left foot*. Los Angeles, CA: Miramax.

van Gennep, A. (1960). *The rites of passage*. London: Routledge and Kegan Paul.

Verbrugge, L. M., and Jette, A. M. (1994). The disablement process. *Social Science and Medicine, 38*(1), 1–14.

Williams. A. (2004). Patients with comorbidities: perceptions of acute care services. *Journal of Advanced Nursing*, 46(1), 13–22.

CHAPTER 12

Transitions in Aging: A Focus on Dementia Care Nursing

Trevor Adams and Wendy Moyle

Overview

The chapter applies Solution-Focused Nursing (SFN) to the work of older people and particularly nurses working with people who have dementia and their family members. Following a discussion of the medical and social processes relating to aging and dementia care, the chapter illustrates these processes through the use of a story. This story describes the experience of a person with dementia (PWD) and challenges various dominant ideas within dementia care nursing. The chapter identifies how nurses may implement SFN and sets it within an inclusive approach towards dementia care that includes the PWD and their family members. Moreover, the chapter argues that it is through different social practices undertaken by the PWD, their family carers and the nurse that knowledge and understanding about what is happening is socially constructed. Through the use of this approach, it is hoped that nurses will be able to develop creative and proactive approaches towards people with dementia and their families that are underpinned by SFN.

Dementia

Dementia is a syndrome which may arise in a number of different conditions such as Alzheimer's disease, Multi-infarct dementia, Parkinson's disease, Alcohol abuse, repeated head injury and infections such as AIDS and Creutzfeldt-Jacob disease (Jacques and Jackson, 2000). Dementia results in the progressive failure of various cerebral functions which interfere with normal cognitive and social functioning, challenges people's sense of self and personhood, and may affect their ability to undertake occupations and activities of daily living. Families often find it difficult to support relatives with dementia and frequently experience considerable stress and burden, which is often the impetus for finding long-term care placement. However, long-term care placement does not always lead to the reduction of stress and burden within family members. Often, long-term care is extremely expensive and places an additional financial burden upon the family and the placement of the person may increase the reality of the loss of a family member (Moyle, Edwards and Clinton, 2002).

Dementia is not a normal part of aging and may develop at any age. Epidemiological studies show that the likelihood of developing dementia rises with age. Between the ages of 65–74 years, it is estimated that the incidence of dementia is about 3% and that at 85 years it is up to 47% (Richter and Richer, 2002). As a result of the increased number of people living over the age of 75 years and also the increased recognition of Alzheimer's disease within the developed world, there is increased risk for dementia.

Different conditions and situations may adversely affect the cognition of older people. Although it is important to first rule out physical causes of presenting clinical features, the dominant biomedical model assumes that changes to emotional or cognitive states are abnormal, must be defined as a medical problem and needs medical treatment. This process is termed 'the medicalization' of behaviours (Estes and Binney, 1989). Because the medical model tends to emphasize the disease process, the person with dementia and their wishes can be overlooked or considered secondary. As a result, their life prospects are constrained or controlled by the medical profession and emphasis is placed on the disease process, while the person themselves are ignored. Medical or psychiatric classification tends to highlight people's abnormalities rather than their strengths (Bond, 2001).

A solution-focused approach helps nurses to overcome undue focus on the diagnosis and instead enables them to implement solution-oriented practice. To enable nurses to set SFN within a wider framework, the approach needs to understand how older people are viewed within society.

Ageism

There is a tendency to think that many older people have Alzheimer's disease whenever they display any emotional change, lose or forget something, or just act eccentrically. Adelman (1995) has identified this phenomenon as 'the Alzheimerization of old age' and raises the issue that the tendency to 'see' older people as having Alzheimer's disease should be resisted by all nurses. It is important to realize that the majority of older people do not have dementia and should not be treated as though they do!

Aging takes place within a social context that exerts various constraints upon older people. It also influences how society views the older people and how nurses provide care. For example, society may encourage older adults to maintain patterns of behaviour that are typical of younger populations. Alternatively, older people may be encouraged to adopt patterns perceived as 'appropriate' to their age or in the case of forgetfulness as outlined above, the older person is labelled with having dementia.

The constraints operating upon older people are numerous and include biological changes that accompany old age as well as social factors such as retirement, the availability of social services, social attitudes, and stereotypes of age-appropriate behaviour in later life. Unfortunately, ageism gives rise to unwarranted discrimination against people on the grounds of age (Butler, 1969), creates its own self-fulfilling prophecies, and promotes lifestyles that damage individual potential. Nurses practice within a framework of personal and professional values. However, these values can influence the attitude of nurses towards aging and affect the provision of quality care. When nurses allow negative beliefs about dementia to affect their practice, it is likely that people with dementia may find themselves discriminated against and marginalized. This stigmatizing process affects how people with dementia feel about themselves. The following story illustrates the social and relational processes that bear down upon the person with dementia and their family within dementia care nursing.

The Jackson's Story

Mr and Mrs Jackson lived in a semi-detached house in a town in the north of England, now part of the conurbation of Greater Manchester. The Consultant Psychiatrist who had visited the couple a few days earlier referred the couple to the Community Mental Health Nurse (CMHN). Mrs Jackson had difficulties with her memory for some time but the Psychiatrist had not fully recognised their extent when he asked Mr Jackson if he could speak to him away from his wife in the kitchen. While they were talking, Mrs Jackson left the house and the Consultant had to get into his car to find her.

Mr Jackson was very committed to looking after his wife. They had married late in life and had no children. They had never been very ill and kept to themselves. Mr Jackson was a quiet man who felt it was his duty to give his wife as much care as she needed. When the CMHN first visited him he had an apron on and was cleaning the kitchen. He told the nurse about his wife's deteriorating health and decline into dementia. His understanding was quite clear and he spoke with concern and compassion about what was happening to his wife. In all that he said, his concern was his wife's welfare. Over the next few visits, an assessment of what current and past happenings was developed. It was very clear that Mrs Jackson was more deteriorated than was at first thought. It seemed that her husband had 'protected' her from being diagnosed and thus as someone who had dementia.

Mr Jackson talked about all the things he was doing for his wife and it was quite clear from what he said that he was exhausted and in need of a break. The CMHN thought that Mrs Jackson needed a place in the day hospital for a few days a week so that Mr Jackson could have a break. However from what

Mr Jackson said, it was clear that he would probably use this time to catch up with the housework.

Reluctantly Mr Jackson said that he would try day care and so it was arranged for Mrs Jackson to attend the day hospital for a daylong assessment. This did not go very well. The ambulance was late and this upset Mrs Jackson and made it difficult for Mr Jackson to get his wife into the ambulance. At the assessment meeting a week later, it was decided to give Mrs Jackson two days a week day care. Mr Jackson politely accepted this offer, though the CMHN accepted upon looking back that his acceptance was reluctant. This gradually became apparent when he insisted on taking and bringing his wife in a taxi to the day hospital. This was financially costly and did not give Mr Jackson enough time to rest at home. After the couple had become familiar with the day hospital and the staff who worked there, the CMHN gradually ceased visiting and all care was handed over.

The CMHN went on to work alongside similar cases with complex needs and it was not until five months later that he heard from the couple again. It was a Friday evening, the end of a busy week. The nurse-in-charge of a long-term care ward phoned to let him know that Mrs Jackson had finally been given a placement. Her husband had suffered a heart attack and was hospitalized, thus leaving no-one to care for his wife. Sadly, a week later the CMHN learned that Mr Jackson died. Within just a few days, so too did his wife.

This story raises difficult questions about the nature of practice within dementia care. Who listens to the voice of the PWD? Who differentiates between the way clinicians see 'the problem' and the way it is seen by the carer? The right for Mrs Jackson to make decisions about her health care was taken from her as her cognitive impairment was seen to restrict her ability to decide what she could or could not do. She had after all 'absconded' from her home. Looking at this in a different light one might say that Mrs Jackson was discriminated against and that stereotypical care, in this case A Day Care Program, was provided based upon her age as well as her disease process, but not perhaps for her personal and family needs.

Reader Activity: There are many transitions we make as we age. Unfortunately sometimes transitional stages involve illness. Recall from your earlier reading what is meant by transitions. Re-read the story and identify transitions that you think Mr and Mrs Jackson may have been experiencing. Compare the transitions that you have documented with the aging section in one of your health care texts.

Dementia Care Nursing and Problem-Centredness

Currently, like many areas of nursing, dementia care nursing tends to be problem-centred rather than solution-focused. Problem-centredness has occurred because dementia care nursing has identified and then used problem-solving, the Nursing Process and Nursing Diagnosis to influence nursing practice.

The Nursing Process is a method for organizing and delivering nursing care. Yura and Walsh (1988) first described the Nursing Process as involving the following three steps:

1. Assessment involving the nurse collecting objective and subjective data in relation to the client's health status,
2. Planning and implementing nursing interventions focused on the client's problem(s), and
3. Evaluation of the effectiveness of the interventions.

'Diagnosis' was later added as a step to be incorporated during assessment planning. Nursing Diagnosis became a recommended and popular practice for nursing from the 1970s to 1990s. But as Powers (2001) has persuasively argued in her critique of nursing diagnosis, the idea of nurses assigning a diagnosis to a patient that is different from a medical diagnosis had the unintended effect of perpetuating a domination over patients, by using the control-based language of science and by approaching the client in terms of their defects. This has the effect, she argues, of placing nurses in a superior position, as one who has both the prescription and the cure and for clients to be seen as the source of the problem.

For many who work in Dementia care, the Nursing Process and Nursing Diagnosis has limited nursing practice to be about reacting to, and intervening in, problems of care. Instead, nurses could be exploring strengths and solutions for health care, whilst also actively involving clients in this process.

We suggest that problem-centredness in aged-care nursing has also been influenced by the overriding dominance of Psychiatry. It was through this speciality, that 'dementia' was first categorised as an organic mental disorder and this has helped to embed its understanding as (nothing but) a problem. While we are not disputing that the medical profession has an important role within health care, we are arguing that the focus on the 'illness as the problem' has meant that the person has tended to be pushed to one side. Normal aging is linked with disease symptoms, encouraging the view within society that the problems of aging need to be defined and treated and that older people are dysfunctional, problematic or of little value. To encourage a positive and effective approach towards the provision of nursing care that focuses on the PWD and their family, we would argue that a solution-focused approach provides an optimistic alternative to problem-centredness.

Solution-Focused Dementia Care Nursing

Besides a medical orientation, or problem-focused approach to dementia care, three other approaches are also emerging as important to dementia care nursing and ought to be considered. The first approach is person-centred care (Kitwood, 1997; Brooker, 2004). This approach highlights the inner subjective experience of people with dementia and constructs people with dementia as having a voice that may, and should, be heard. An important feature of this approach is that people with dementia are seen as possessing personhood and that this state is bestowed them through the interaction they have with other people. In this way, person-centred care may be seen as highlighting the importance of relationships and the relational nature of dementia care.

Reader Activity: Reflect on the case study. Write down the dominant voice in the decision making for Mrs Jackson. Whose voices are not heard? What do you think they would say?

The second approach highlights the rise of the community as carer in which family members and informal carers such as volunteers and lifestyle assistants are recruited to help and support the person with dementia so that they can live in the community for as long as possible (Forbat, 2005; Heaton, 1999). Although a community-oriented approach has obvious strengths, it also has deficits. One consequence is that diverse and sometimes disconnected services focusing on the PWD or their informal carer have developed. One example in the United Kingdom is the 'Admiral Nursing Service' which develops nurses to work within domiciliary dementia care settings and identifies their first objective quite clearly as to 'work with family carers as their prime focus' http://www.fordementia.org.uk/admiral.htm, accessed 12 April 2005). The implication is that the Admiral Nursing Service privileges the voice and concerns of family carers and may marginalize the person with dementia.

Recently various attempts have been made to develop a model of integrated care, where the PWD, their informal carer, and the dementia care nurse work together. Keady (1999) describes how people with dementia and their informal carers undertake the process of 'working together' as they come to terms and address difficulties that have arisen as a result of the development of dementia. There is also potential to add to that working group, the family as well as relevant social groups.

This approach was initially developed in the United States by Silliman (1989) and has been incorporated within various models such as the 'partnership approach' (Adams, 1999), 'triadic interaction' (Fortinsky, 2001), and 'relationship centred care' (Nolan *et al.*, 2004; Keady and Nolan, 2003). The underlying idea within these approaches is that dementia care is often provided within 'dementia care triads'[1] comprising the PWD, the informal carer(s), and

[1] The term 'dementia care triad' is used to refer to groups consisting of a person with dementia, one or more family carers, and one or more health and social care practitioners. Often though, dementia care triads comprise three people – the person with dementia, the primary family carer, and the dementia care nurse.

one or more health and social care professional. While the triad is often the focus of counselling, there are often other family members and health and social care professionals who contribute to the provision of care (Keith, 1995).

Integrated care acknowledges that there are sometimes complex interplays between the various members of the working group. Adams (2002) has argued that alliances and coalitions often develop within dementia care triads so that two triad members may align to form a coalition and leave the third member isolated, disempowered and marginalized.

In the context of solution-focused nursing, dementia care nurses us different approaches within practice. Solution-focused approaches provide nurses with an opportunity to enable PWD and their family to reframe identities and practice settings. It also facilitates the generation of innovative solutions by building on the strengths, achievements, and capacity of PWD and their family.

Theory into Practice

But how is that done? How can you make the transition from problem-centred nursing to solution-focused nursing? As indicated above there are several approaches that have developed within nursing and more specifically within dementia care nursing. These approaches however still may focus on the individual, rather than the individual's problems. Solution-focused nursing as an alternative approach focuses on building solutions rather than concentrating on problem solving. If we reflect on the story of Mr and Mrs Jackson we can see that little attention was given to the voice of Mrs Jackson, and Mr Jackson needs were decided for him, perhaps in this case because of his age and increasing frailty. We know that stories such as the Jackson's, where both family members are aging and one has a dementing illness, are not uncommon and so we need to consider how best to address these.

If we were to recreate or 're-story' this story and use a SFN approach to care management this would mean that we would:

1. Incorporate the voice of the PWD and their family carer in decisions about their care;
2. Remind health professionals of the importance of working alongside the PWD and their family carer rather than just focusing on the disease process;
3. Listen and respect the views and opinions of the PWD and their carer;
4. Try to see the emergence of solutions rather than just problems;
5. Build on the strengths of the PWD and their carer so that they feel involved in the management of care and can own and see positive aspects of their role and position with the care setting;

6. Accept the symptoms and behaviours that may arise as a result of the dementing process rather than seeing them as problems that must be treated;
7. If the family carer believes they can manage, and when it appears that they are having difficulty coping with the situation, work alongside them to develop strategies that will make their life easier, rather than take their role away from them;
8. Look at how the PWD interacts with people, environment and treatments and explore, trial and implement alternative solutions that may improve their quality of life;
9. Introduce meaning with a focus on personhood, which accommodates the view of the world held by the PWD;
10. Help the PWD and their carer identify social networks that will be act as source of support and a form of social capital.

Conclusion

This chapter has discussed the contribution of different approaches within health care and Dementia Care Nursing in particular. The chapter argues that being solution-focused within dementia care nursing needs to include not just on the PWD but also should include informal carers, family, other social groups and nurses. In addition, the chapter challenged traditional approaches within dementia care nursing. We argued for, and showed how, Solution-focused nursing represents an opportunity to acknowledge feelings and behaviours that are part of an individual and social experience of dementia, and to develop creative and imaginative ways of providing effective solutions to dementia care issues.

Reader Activity: Reflect on the strategies outlined above and the case study presented of Mr and Mrs Jackson and write down how you might use SFN to manage this situation more effectively.

Suggestions for Further Reading

Adams, T., and Manthorpe, J. (2003). *Dementia care.* London: Arnold.

Draper, B. (2004). *Dealing with dementia. A guide to Alzheimer's disease and other dementias.* Crows Nest, New South Wales: Allen and Unwin.

Dunne, R. (2002). *Dementia care programming: an identity-focused approach*, New York: Venture Press.

References

Adelman, R. (1995). The Alzheimerisation of aging. *Gerontologist, 35*(4), 526–532.

Bond, J. (2001). Sociological perspectives. Ch. 3. In C. Cantley (ed.). *A handbook of dementia care.*(pp. 44–61). Buckingham: Open University Press.

Burr, V. (2003). *An introduction to social constructionism (2nd Ed.).*London: Routledge.

Butler, R. (1969). Ageism. Another form of bigotry. *Gerontologist, 9*, 243–246.

Estes, C.L. and Binney, E. (1989). The biomedicalisation of aging: dangers and dilemmas. *Gerontologist, 29* (5), 587–596.

Heaton, J. (1999). The gaze and visibility of the carer: a Foucauldian analysis of the discourse of informal care. *Sociology of Health and Illness*, 21, 759–777.

Forbat, L. (2005). *Talking about care – two sides to the story.* Bristol: Policy Press.

Jacques, A. and Jackson, G. (2000). *Understanding dementia. 3rd ed.* Edinburgh: Churchill Livingstone.

Moyle. W., Edwards, H., and Clinton, M. (2002). Living with loss: Dementia and the family caregiver. *Australian Journal of Advanced Nursing, 19* (3), 25–31.

Powers, P. (2001). A discourse analysis of nursing diagnosis. Chapter 4 in P.Powers. *The methodology of discourse analysis* (pp.67–138). Boston, MA: Jones and Bartlett.

Ritcher, R. W. and Ritcher, B. (2002). *Alzheimer's disease.* St Louis: Mosby.

Yura, H. and Walsh, M. (1988). *The nursing process, 5th ed.* New York: Appleton-Century-Crofts.

CHAPTER 13

Facilitating Family, Friends and Community Transition Through the Experience of Loss

Paul Morrison

Overview

> Dealing with our grief, with all the losses we have experienced, is not about moving on and forgetting. It's about remembering our people and bringing them with us wherever we go (Wingard, 2001)

Death is another life transition, wherein nurses have a key role in facilitating peoples' adaptation, acceptance and successful resolution. Even though it may seem obvious that during this time many problems such as pain, immobility, fear, and discomfort need to be managed, a solution orientation can also offer nurses skills in being person-focused, motivating, connecting and life-affirming. There are many interpersonal and technical skills that need to be mastered. The author provides stories of sudden loss and expected loss and discusses how the nurse's approach within it was solution focused.

Introduction

The therapeutic practice of nurses has never been clearly articulated and this facet of nursing has, I fear, been more imagined than real except in a most rudimentary sense. These days there is a great need to expand the therapeutic role of the nurse. There may be many ways to do this but I believe that some of the ideas outlined in this chapter offer a very interesting path; a path that can lead to the creation of a brighter landscape for nursing by expanding the helping focus in our work.

The chapter starts with a story about the grief and loss experienced by Orla and Fergus and at the same time tells the story of some of the therapy choices, paths and considerations that have influenced my own work as a nurse and a psychologist. Instead of advocating the merits of a particular school or approach, I have found it more helpful to focus on the aspects and ideas in my own work that I revisit constantly. These help me to work with people to find solutions to the difficulties in their lives.

The chapter will therefore include some discussion on the need to place our work in a particular historical context, to strive for enhanced self-awareness, to be clear about our beliefs about people and helping and to work in ways that feel right for you and me. As the chapter unfolds, I hope that you will see how these ideas may be used to help people like Orla and Fergus.

The Story

At the age of 33, Orla who is now 48 moved to Australia from Ireland. She had a successful nursing career and was very happy, although having been raised in a catholic Irish community, yearned to meet a man and begin a family. Five years earlier, Fergus, who is now 50, had also emigrated to Australia from Ireland. He worked as a carpenter, and he too longed to make a family. But being hard working folk they did not have much time for relationships and marriage and had begun to feel resigned to the idea that they might never marry or have children.

But as luck would have it, Orla and Fergus were introduced at a mutual friend's BBQ and immediately struck up a rapport. They fell in love and married. They were obviously 'made for each other' and rekindled their shared hope of having children. Their sisters and brothers on both sides of the family had each produced a number of children. Then, after two years of trying, Orla and Fergus were about to give up on the idea of babies, when Orla found herself pregnant. Kilian's birth was the realization of a dream for both Orla and Fergus and they lived happily in Brisbane, Queensland.

At eight years of age Kilian was doing well at school, he had a group of very good friends and followed the Brisbane Broncos with fanatical zeal. He had a season ticket and went to all the home games with his parents. He and his parents were planning a trip to Ireland during the summer break to coincide with Kilian's ninth birthday and they were all looking forward to meeting up with their extended family and the 'craic' in Ireland during the northern hemisphere Christmas. But Kilian did not make it to Ireland that year. He died two weeks before Christmas Day after a short period in hospital for the treatment of a high-grade astrocytoma (brain tumour).

Ten months after Kilian's death Orla and Fergus were still heartbroken and in great pain – so much so that they felt they could not continue to live in this state of 'constant heartache'. Their friends and families were a great support initially and reassured them that 'time would heal their hearts' but it didn't seem to make any real difference in their lives. Kilian was gone and the happiness they found together which was cemented with the arrival of Kilian was ruptured irretrievably and they feared now that their own relationship might come asunder ...

The Context of Grief-Work

When we think about the word solution or having a solution focus in our work as professional helpers there may well be a tendency to slip into 'fix-it' mode. Many professional helpers and nurses in particular, have an inclination to want to fix things including peoples' pain following traumatic life events and illnesses. The desire to help and to fix is an admirable one and one which needs to be acknowledged. However, it places the helper in a position of power and expertise that is not warranted nor is it likely to be helpful.

A solution-focused approach can also be considered as a process of helping others to find *their own* answers, responses, or ways of acknowledging the realities of their lives. It can also mean that people find an acceptable interpretation of life events that fits with their preferred identities and values or that they find a sense of completion with these events and happenings. Adapting a solution-focused approach in your work can mean much more than applying a quick fix.

However, in the traditional and current climate of health care, many health professionals tend to focus on the goals of the institution rather than the goals and needs of those who seek their help. A major emphasis of this orientation is driven by the discipline of medicine and this is not all that surprising given that medicine has had a pre-eminent role in the development of health services and the hierarchical structures that can be found within and across settings.

Moreover, the hub of much nursing work has been aligned with the achievement of institutional and medically driven goals and this has curtailed the potential therapeutic role of nurses. It has limited their capacity to shape their work towards the needs of patients and families in creative and non-pathologising ways. This is not to say that what has occurred historically is wrong; but I think it is time to look towards other ways of working with people that have a non-medical emphasis.

Consider for a moment how death, loss and grief have been treated in the professional health literature. In a commentary on the prevailing attitudes to death and dying in Western societies, Kübler-Ross (1981) stated that: 'the more we are achieving advances in science, the more we seem to fear and deny the reality of death' (p. 6). This is clear from the language we use when talking about death and dying as it conveys our attitudes and cultural mores on the matter and often attempts to negate the reality of death.

This is not so in other societies where death is accepted as part of the natural cycle of life. Nevertheless, Worden (1991) argues that despite cultural differences, and individual reactions to death and dying, a common theme is that we all wish to regain the lost person and a belief that we will meet the dead person in some form of afterlife.

Thus the professional context of care provides a setting for our practice that is, in the main, somewhat austere and traditional. It is important to reflect on this context of care from time to time to be clear about your preferred position and ways of working with people and to limit some of the negative aspects of this care context.

Reader Activity: Take a moment or two and reflect on the ways in which dying people and their families have been cared for in some of the clinical areas you have worked. Share these in class with fellow students. What conclusions emerge?

Reader Activity: Consider the following questions and your reactions to these events:
Have you ever been to a funeral or a wake?
Have you seen a dead person in your clinical work?
Have any of your friends lost a close relative?
Has someone close to you died in the last couple of years?
How have any of these experiences influenced you views or values?

First Things First – Do Your Own Work

The approaches I tend to use have been influenced by my personal history and professional experience and this is something that a good professional helper can use in their work. However, it requires self-awareness, which needs to be developed and nurtured constantly and conscientiously (Burnard, 2002). You need to become more aware of your strengths, weaknesses, wishes, intentions, values and so on.

I am reminded all the time, how my work experience in nursing, psychology, and education, in Ireland, UK, and Australia and my exposure to diverse cultures and peoples, has helped me to become more accepting of diversity and change. These experiences have, I believe, helped to make me a more effective professional.

Striving for enhanced self-awareness reminds me that I belong to a particular race with a particular social history (strong Irish Catholic upbringing) and speak English with a particular type of accent. It also helps me to be aware that *every* client will have his or her own cultural and personal history just like me. However, the process of developing self-awareness is an ongoing one as the challenges in life and work are forever changing, but it is essential to be able to tune in to the other person's world in a non-judgemental way.

Reader Activity: Identify three facets of your own make-up that might limit your capacity to be non-judgemental when caring for recently bereaved people.

The Person-Centred Approach as a Basis For Helping

The person-centred approach to helping was greatly influenced by Carl Rogers (1961). I think this approach to helping provides a very sound basis and orientation for any form of helping or specific approach to therapy. The optimistic outlook of human nature within this approach means that the beneficial process of change that occurs is fashioned by the client not the nurse.

A positive atmosphere may be developed when the nurse displays three key attributes:

1. Congruence, or genuineness
2. Unconditional positive regard, meaning provision of acceptance and care and,
3. Empathic understanding of the subjective world and experience of the client (Corey, 1996).

The assumption is that everyone has the potential to resolve his or her worries. The nurse's role primarily is one of supporting the person to do this by enabling them to renew their knowledge and appreciation for abilities and competencies that they may have lost sight of.

The nurse may help the client to detect their own goals in therapy by establishing a trusting helping relationship with clients and creates a climate in which the client feels safe to explore their self-perceptions and experience a range of feelings. Person-centred helping emphasizes development and in various ways takes some of the obscurity from therapeutic interactions. Rogers stated that: 'psychotherapy is the releasing of an already existing capacity in a potentially competent individual' (1959, p.221). Hence the client holds the keys to solving their struggles while the helper's role is one of assisting in this venture with support and understanding.

In terms of Orla and Fergus, we can make use of a person-centred approach to build a good rapport by listening attentively with an empathic and respectful manner and exploring the significant personal loss in their lives, a type of loss all of us must face at some point in our lives. The death of a person we know and love is perhaps the most painful loss that most people will experience and can be quite devastating.

Being there for Orla and Fergus – spending time with them and helping to talk about the role that Kilian played in their lives, will help them to express strong and painful emotions. This may be a very emotional time for us as nurses too, with awkward feelings of not knowing what to say.

However, being there and listening carefully will be of great value; trying to be a 'companion' and 'walk alongside' Orla and Fergus in a 'meaningful relationship' (Geldard, 1998) as they recount the awful sadness in their lives. The person-centred ideas are I believe, quite indispensable for the approaches I will cover next. I mention them here to ensure that they are not forgotten.

Group Activity: Take a few moments to think about someone in your family (or social network) who has been a positive influence in your life but who has passed away (it could be a teacher, friend, grandparent and so on). In what ways did they change your life? What was it about your relationship with them that you want to take with you into your future live and work? Discuss in the group.

Narrative Therapy meets Solution-Focused Nursing

An approach that I have found increasingly valuable is narrative therapy; it is more a philosophy or belief system than a set of techniques that can be learned and honed with experience (White and Epston, 1990). My interest in narrative ideas grew from a general sense of dissatisfaction with a lot of things I'd learned and experienced in nursing and psychology, together with a growing interest in people and the social context of their lives. When I came across narrative practice I immediately felt at home. The ideas resonated with me as a person and a professional helper.

After attending a number of intensive training programs at the Dulwich Centre in Adelaide, which were facilitated by Michael White, who is one of the leading writers in this area, and meeting with participants from all over the world, I was helped to shape my preferred ways of working with people and the problems they experience. Narrative practice focusses on listening to, and encouraging, stories from people and the problems in their lives. It uses a conversational format and aims to help people shape new realities and identities for themselves.

This orientation, like solution-focused nursing, is founded on a number of important beliefs. To begin with, the person is not the problem, the problem is the problem. This can be quite a tricky notion to work with as much of our training and experience as nurses encourages us to locate problems within individuals. Working with a problem as separate and externalized from the person (for example, exploring the impact of the grief, the pain, the heartache on peoples' lives) opens up spaces to clients to see the problem differently.

Next, people construct meaning around the dominant storylines or narratives in their lives and live their lives accordingly. The role of the therapist is one of helping clients to explore the meanings in their life and helping them to tell a different story of themselves. Clients are the 'experts' on their own lives, the therapist is not.

The helper adopts a stance of genuine curiosity about the client's life, which entails asking questions you (the nurse) do not know the answer to. Detailed and very readable accounts of narrative ideas can be found elsewhere (see for example Morgan, 2000).

Re-storying lives is of value not just for individuals, but also for groups in society. (2001) described how 'talking together' and sharing stories of family losses within an Aboriginal context highlights some of the cultural aspects of grief and loss that may go unrecognized:

> A lot of Aboriginal people also experience signs from loved ones who have passed away. Seeing particular birds, for example, is often experienced as having ongoing contact with people who have died, ongoing contact with their spirits (p. 2).

It's worth noting too that those who don't understand the cultural context, could perceive such signs as examples of pathology.

Rethinking Grief Work

The application of narrative ideas in relation to grief has been beautifully illustrated in the book 'Remembering Practices' (Hedkte and Winslade, 2004). The authors note that in Western settings many of the conversations we have about death and dying use language, which emphasizes the finality of death and the end of relationships by seeking closure, moving on, saying good-bye and letting go. These are all examples of the widespread view this is what occurs in a normal grieving process.

However they argue that these sorts of conversations may well render the grieving process more painful and unbearable. Hedke and Winslade (2004) go on to suggest that our memories of the lost loved ones often rekindle their role in our current and futures lives and the influence they have had and may continue to have when we invite them into our lives. This view forms the basis of remembering conversations, which can provide great comfort to grieving people.

Remembering conversations makes it possible to provide comfort and add to peoples' lives, not by dwelling on their pain, but by embracing the dead in the lives of the living. The focus is on honouring their contributions to the lives of others. This notion helps people to deal with the death of someone close in a very non-traditional way by bringing new hope to those grieving. Hopes that help sustain them now and into the future by ensuring that the dead person continues to be an important part of their lives and identities.

There is a wonderfully moving account of similar narrative work with a family who lost their daughter through suicide in Michael White's book on folk psychology (2001). Drawing on aspects of this account we might begin the following conversation with Orla and Fergus:

> I am curious to learn more about how your lives are changed for having Kilian as a son. I have a sense that it made your lives different in terms of how you yourselves think and act today that are a testimony to his short life. Perhaps you might share with me some of those life-changing stories.

This kind of invitation provides a basis for generating new accounts or conversations about Kilian's contribution to their lives. It might help Orla and Fergus to talk about the gifts that Kilian gave them: fun, excitement, energy, exuberance, joy and deep, unconditional love. Remembering these gifts are his legacy to Orla and Fergus and indeed to others who knew and were touched by him.

These conversations can evoke, crystallize and capture memories that grieving people will want to take with them and cherish in their own future lives. They can help ensure that Kilian continues to play a critical role in Fergus and Orla's lives in ways that are sustaining and enriching of their lives.

Similarly, Wingard (2001) described how 'gatherings' within Aboriginal communities provide ways of helping people remember the lost loved one in ways that make the participants in the gathering stronger in their own lives. Hedtke and Winslade (2004) argue that this type of remembering practice has a healing and inspiring effect on those grieving.

Orla and Fergus need to feel heard and understood and their great loss acknowledged and validated. A little later we could ask questions like: How did you get through this last month, or year? How did you manage to keep going? Where did you get the strength to make it though this? These questions will generate ideas about coping and surviving. They may also open up opportunities for conversations, which include Kilian and how he has helped them to get through this awful time in their lives.

Possibilities for the future can be explored when a basis for coping has been established. This future focus can help Orla and Fergus to 'construct their own solutions, which is a key to being brief and successful with any presenting problem' (Butler and Powers, 1996, p. 231).

Another approach here is to look for exceptions that emphasize coping: 'How do you keep it from getting worse? How do you keep it together and go to work everyday?' These sorts of questions will acknowledge the struggle that Orla and Fergus have been through and reinforce the actions they have taken or the strengths they found within themselves and used to keep things from getting worse.

There is another facet of the solution-focused approach that may be used effectively here which raises possibilities for the future. You could use scaling questions as these may have the effect of focusing Orla and Fergus onto specific actions they might take in the near future (Butler and Powers, 1996): 'On a scale of one to ten, where one is the worst this has been, and ten is the best things could ever be, where are things today?' (O'Hanlon and Weiner-Davis, 1989).

If Orla and Fergus indicated that they were at two on the scale, then this could be followed up with a question on the signs that might indicate that they were moving towards two and a half or a three. Their answers can then be expanded on and in so doing Orla and Fergus could map out the specific ways in which they can move in a preferred direction. Even small increments of movements along a preferred direction can be expanded on in conversation and help move the couple towards some form of resolution for their grief.

The process of story-telling, identifying gifts left behind, using rituals or gatherings, and questions that search for exceptions and scale change may help sustain the relationship and foster hope rather than prematurely stop them. These strategies can assist people to deal with grief in quite different and life enhancing ways (Hedkte and Winsalde, 2004).

Group Activity: Divide into pairs (A and B) and take turns with this exercise. 'A' briefly describes a time in their life when things were difficult. It does not have to be too draining emotionally and could include times when you failed an assignment and thought about leaving the course, or the budgie died or a time when you were so broke you could not afford to pay the telephone bill. 'B' listens attentively, demonstrates curiosity and encourages 'A' to tell the story fully and then asks 'How did you keep it from getting worse? How did you keep it together and go to work everyday?'. B encourages A to expand on these.
Reverse the roles.
Feedback to the larger group on the experience of completing the exercise.

Conclusion

Dealing with death, dying and caring for those who are grieving is a normal part of life for all of us. As a nurse however, you will have to face this area of work and its repercussions frequently and as you get older in your personal life too. Sometimes nursing presents the personal heartache and distress that occurs in other peoples' lives to very young students. When it does, it can occur in a forceful and shocking manner and at the most unexpected times.

At the end of the day, you will need to manage the emotional turmoil and responses to these life events in yourself and others. If you don't, your work may become unbearable instead of challenging, revitalizing and rewarding. Learning to deal effectively with these inevitable aspects of life and respond confidently through enhanced self-awareness, the development of specialist counselling skills and increased cultural sensitivity, will enhance your professional functionality and help you remain fit and well personally.

If applied sensibly and thoughtfully, the approaches mentioned here have the potential to endow nurses with some very powerful ideas for practice no matter where they work. Many nurses with a desire to become more therapeutic in their practice will tend to take an eclectic approach or one that is influenced by a few schools or theories instead of relying on just one framework. Such an approach is very sensible.

However, the key to unlocking your real potential as a professional helper is to find a way of working that fits with the person you are and strive to be, one that is closely aligned with the values and beliefs you hold dear. The ideas sketched in this chapter could become a rich and rewarding vein of discovery for the intrepid explorer.

Suggestions for Further Reading

Hedtke, L. and Winslade, J. (2004). *Re-membering lives: conversations with the dying and the bereaved.* New York: Baywood, Amityville.

Milner, J. and O'Byrne, P. (2002). *Brief counselling: narratives and solutions.* Basingstoke: Palgrave.

Morgan, A. (2000). *What is narrative therapy. An easy-to-read introduction.* Adelaide: Dulwich Centre.

Payne, M. (2000). *Narrative therapy: An introduction for counsellors.* London: Sage.

Teacher notes to accompany this chapter can be found at www.palgrave.com/nursinghealth/mcallister

References

Burnard, P. (2002). *Learning human skills. An experiential and reflective guide for nurses.* 4th edition. London: Butterwork-Heinemann.

Butler, W. and Powers, K. (1996). Solution-focused grief therapy. In: S.D Miller, M.A. Hubble, B. L. Duncan, (eds), *Handbook of solution-focused brief therapy.* (pp. 228–247). San Francisco, CA: Jossey-Bass.

Corey, G. (1996). *Theory and practice of counselling and psychotherapy.* 5th edition, Pacific Grove: Brooks/Cole.

Geldard, D. (1998). *Basic counselling skills.* 3rd edition, Australia, Prentice Hall.

Hedtke, L. and Winslade, J. (2004). *Re-membering lives: conversations with the dying and the bereaved.* New York, Baywood.

O'Hanlon, W. and Weiner-Davis, M. (1989). *In search of solution.* New York, Norton.

Rogers, C. (1959). A theory of therapy, personality and interpersonal relationships, as developed in the client-centred framework. In: S. Koch (ed.), *Psychology: a study of a science.* Vol. 3, New York, McGraw-Hill, pp. 184–256.

Rogers, C.R. (1961). *On becoming a person.* Boston, LA: Houghton Mifflin.

White, M. (2001). *Folk psychology and narrative practice.* Dulwich Centre Journal, 2, 3–17.

White, M. and Epston, D. (1990). *Narrative means to therapeutic ends.* Adelaide, Dulwich Centre Publications.

Wingard, B. (2001). *Telling our stories in ways that make us stronger.* Adelaide, Dulwich Centre Publications. *Accessed on the internet on 09/05/05 at www.dulwichcentre.com.au/*

Worden, J. (1991). *Grief counselling and grief therapy.* 2nd edition, London, Routledge.

CHAPTER 14

Helping Other People to be Solution-Focused

Margaret McAllister

Growth and New Beginnings

I'm imagining that you are by now an informed reader of Solution-Focused Nursing. In my mind's eye I can see that you have a solid idea of the tenets of SFN and know that it is a subtle, yet profound, step beyond other approaches to health care provision that are problem-focused. You've examined the cultural roots within health care, nursing and society that help to keep people preoccupied with problems, rather than motivated towards change. You can appreciate the value in systematic problem-solving and can use these skills to perform a competent and respectful assessment of a client. You have exercised your creativity and know to use both imaginative and rational reasoning in your nursing work.

The challenge ahead will be to find ways to keep those creative juices flowing and to maintain a commitment to being solution oriented even when the environment around you may tend towards problems and trouble-talk. Being somewhat of a renegade will be a risky and at times lonely adventure, but you are not alone. History is full of courageous individuals and groups who were determined to change the system, and you can learn from them.

Reader Activity: Read the lyrics of the Indigo Girls' song entitled 'Hammer and a Nail' (2000). [It would be even better if you can listen to the music, because something of the emotion, emphasis and meaning can be lost when a song is reduced to its words.]
Consider its application to nursing by completing this activity:

1. What opinion is the song expressing?
2. Now work out what you think an opposing point of view could be.
3. Decide which point of view has the most value.
4. In what ways can you see the ideas of this song to be of relevance to nursing.

I hope that reading these chapters has been challenging and stimulated you to think about practices in new ways. I invite you now to take time to think about your future practice, and to imagine new beginnings.

Hammer and a nail, by the Indigo Girls

I had a lot of good intentions
Sit around for fifty years
And then collect a pension
Started seeing the road to hell
And just where it starts
But my life is more than a vision
The sweetest part is acting
After making a decision
Started seeing the whole
As a sum of its parts
(Chorus) And I look behind my ears for the green
And even my sweat smells clean
Glare off the white hurts my eyes
Gotta get out of bed
Get a hammer and a nail
Learn how to use my hands
Not just my head
I think myself in a jail
Now I know a refuge never grows
From a chin in a hand
And a thoughtful pose
Gotta tend the earth
If you want a rose
My life is part of the global life
I'd found myself becoming more immobile
When I'd think a little girl in the world
Can't do anything
A distant nation my community
And a street person my responsibility
If I have a care in the world
I have a gift to bring

My students, friends and colleagues have said to me that an important insight about SFN that they take from this song is the belief in *committed action*. This is a concept that recurs throughout this book and is also important to critical theorists working in education, research and social work. SFN and critical theory share the view that ideas are only as good as the actions that lead from them. This song can remind us also that SFN is not just concerned with the health and well-being of individuals but also with communities, for these are inextricably linked and influence each other. There are likely to be many more lessons embedded within this song, perhaps you could use this medium or something similar to generate imaginative solutions from your friends, colleagues and future clients.

Learning from the Wisdom of Others

This song is also about staying grounded in your own values. Recently, I asked students and colleagues I have known to share strategies they found useful in keeping them true to their beliefs. With their permission I convey them now to you so that you can benefit from their wisdom and do not have to be alone in your struggle to stay committed to ideals. I have organized their comments around contexts in which the pressure to conform, or let go of ideals, seem to be at their greatest.

At Handover

Handover can be a very testing time for solution focused nurses because it is the place where dominant discourses are most prominently revealed. Parker *et al.*, (1992) argued that nurses engage in a kind of *silencing* in handovers. That is, there are things about clients that are not said for some reason. They also argue that what nurses have to say about clients in other forums, such as in team meetings, is being silenced by others and by themselves.

If you practice within a non-mainstream, less conventional practice paradigm, then you may find yourself and your beliefs being silenced or sanctioned in this environment.

Reader Activity: Recall the skills learned in chapter 3. Use that knowledge to think of a recent 'ward round' or 'team meeting' and analyse it using dialectical thinking. In what ways do nurses speak of their work within the medical model? Then, on the other hand, in what ways do they also talk about the client's growing resilience and recovery?

Craig Shepperd, a nurse unit manager agreed that handover time can be challenging:

> In handover, it is especially easy to fall into the trap of communicating in a medical type framework. This is because we primarily focus on illness and problems rather than the client and solutions, strength and positives.
>
> One of the ways that I try to keep it nurse-focused is through the use of the nursing process. I present subjective and objective information about the client, my

> assessment(s) throughout the shift, the nursing plan developed, the interventions we used and how well they worked.
>
> I think another important way I keep nurse-focused (which is also being client-focused) is through the language I use. For example, I avoid terms that use the illness as the descriptive factor. Instead of saying 'Mr Jones is a 32 year old Diabetic' I may say something along the lines of 'Mr Jones is a 32 year old man who is currently experiencing neuropathy. He has a history of Diabetes' In this way, I'm trying to put the person and their needs before their diagnosis.

When being with Clients

Another important context, which seems so obvious, but which is often a place that is kept hidden from public view, is the nurse–client relationship. If we were to think more consciously about what gets lived out in this encounter, and what clients as members of the general public come to learn about nursing, we might see this as an extremely important place to make an impression and to show how nursing can be more than illness-oriented, and more solution-focused.

John Haberecht, a palliative care nurse and President of the Holistic Nurses Association in Australia, explained his approach:

> It's very much about therapeutic use of self, something that we generally do unconsciously I think, but which is extremely powerful. In my work it's about taking the time to be with clients and families, letting them know that I'm there for them, and that they can contact our team even after hours if there's a significant problem.
>
> But it's more than just that practical assistance, it's a way of being with people that can be hard to articulate – it's the way that you walk into the room and are there with them so that your body language indicates that you're not about to rush off to the next patient, or thinking about the numerous other tasks you have to do.
>
> It's also communicated in your eye contact, your facial expression, tone of voice – all those things that are so much a part of who we are as a person and which communicate that to our clients very powerfully whether we like it or not. We can mouth the words and the platitudes, but if we're not being genuine, they'll see through us straight away.
>
> I believe this is what nursing is about at its essence – the nurse seeing the client as a whole and coming from a place of honouring the client as a whole human being.

During Trouble Talk

It's not just nurses, but the whole of society it seems, who like to engage in talking about what's going wrong with the world. But trouble-talk is problem-focused and is really a way for us all to remain locked in to old ways of imagining the world. Trouble talk is unlikely to be optimistic and unlikely to offer creative ways of re-thinking life's problems.

Beth Matarasso spoke about ways she gently models to her colleagues ways of staying person-focused and resisting the temptation to always talk about what's going wrong.

> When I first engage with a client, I am keen to get to know them – what they like to do, what they read, basically what their life is like. One young woman that I know can be difficult to engage sometimes, she can be a bit regressed, acts like a 13 year old. But during election time we engaged in some great discussions about politics and this literally makes her shine.
>
> I shared this with a colleague who was describing their difficulty with engaging her and she told me that on their next encounter she engaged her in this way to open her up and it worked beautifully and has provided a basis for them to know each other.

These stories, separately and together, offer lessons for those who are ready to listen. I wonder if you can work out what those common themes are. Creativity, imagination and focusing on strengths not problems are also important cognitive processes (see Table 14.1 for more ideas).

Table 14.1 Creative strategies for staying focused on SFN in practice

1. Gently question yours and others' myths that have become taken-for-granted
2. Reject negative images of nursing and health care
3. Be proud and claim your caring traditions in practice as being valuable, unique contributions to social health and well-being
4. Limit opportunities for trouble-talk, and instead talk about achievements and ideas
5. Contribute to the enrichment of nursing's culture by publicly applauding
6. All our courageous leaders, joining in rituals and celebrations that unite us
7. Become a producer of new media stories about nursing and not just a consumer
8. Be an advocate of Quality Education programs to build nurses' knowledge and skills
9. Notice and value everyday work, even that which is mundane for the difference it makes in humanizing health care services
10. When you come across a seemingly insoluble problem, reframe it
11. Focus on 'Being with' clients, as well as 'doing for'
12. Be proactive about building healthy spaces for clients and society
13. Be proactive at all health levels: with the client, with each other, and in society

Strategies for Staying Focused in SFN Education

People working as teachers, academics, or researchers in universities are lucky to be surrounded by students new to nursing. Students often have the fresh eyes needed to look at health services anew, to raise challenging questions and to invent new ways of caring. But they are also fragile and rely on a stable, safe learning environment to sustain their passions. It's not enough for educators to mother students for they are not children. It's also not sufficient to simply guide.

Teachers have a responsibility to use their creativity, expertise and technical resources to do more than deliver information. Good teaching is about informative interaction. In nursing, it means showing students how to nurse and how to *be* a nurse. The question is how do educators approach this challenge? It may be helpful to look outside ourselves for answers.

In primary and secondary schools there is an ever-present concern about students' literacy. Rather than discuss reading, writing and arithmetic, there is now talk about developing multiple literacies in students (Cummins and Sayers, 1999): learning how to navigate and communicate through the internet, email, mobile phones, video and television media; learning how to comprehend texts as well as to read and write fluently and finally, learning how to go beneath surface meaning to understand the deep meaning of events and processes. In addition to this media literacy, there is also emphasis on developing students' emotional literacy, multi-cultural literacy and social literacy. How do teachers manage?

I asked Jamie Hay, an experienced high school teacher about the challenge of teaching Shakespeare to 16 year olds.

> The idea is to get students to see the value in it, and do things that show the connection between literature and life. It's good to start by asking students what they don't like about Shakespeare and typically they'll say they don't understand it. They say it's boring, things like that. And then I might challenge those myths by showing an exciting part of Baz Luhrman's Romeo and Juliet.
>
> I usually spend some time talking about and showing how I would interpret key concepts in the play. I then set a task for students to practise the skills I have just modeled, which requires them to transform ideas from one form to another. For example, I might ask students to write a newspaper story about the brawl that happens in the opening scenes. This task requires students to find meaning in the play and then to put that meaning into their own words and language.
>
> We continue to practise these interpretation/translation skills and then I would assess students by having them demonstrate that learning has occurred. I think it is important when setting assessment activities that it be something that is itself a learning experience. I'm really conscious that I don't want the task to simply be a way of training students in how to complete exams. So it needs to be engaging, relevant and connected to the subject under inquiry and to life.

The message that I take from this approach is that it is important to find out where students are at, engage them, spend time in showing how to interpret, translate and connect texts to everyday life, and then give students opportunity to practice and demonstrate learning. For teachers of Solution-Focused Nursing, these strategies have resonance.

The big idea of Solution-focused nursing is to reveal dominant discourses and open them up to scrutiny, debate and perhaps revision so that students of nursing become critically aware rather than passive supporters of the status quo. Within this overarching goal are objectives or learning outcomes specific to a course. Just as there is no single way students of nursing can approach being solution-focused with clients, there is no one way to teach. Indeed, creativity and multiplicity is enriching. (See Table 14.2, which outlines a structure for being solution focused in the classroom.)

In order to generate a culture of sharing and pride in the craft of teaching nursing, I can suggest a number of ways (see Table 14.1) to approach the work of teaching differently. Taking the time to discuss teaching strategies with colleagues and making a concerted attempt to devise left- and right-brained activities may be useful. Because SFN emphasizes creative ways of knowing as well as logic and reason, you may find that re-reading some of the chapters in this book gives you more novel ideas to use. Feel free to use the stories too. Table 14.2 also outlines some ways of staying solution-focused within the classroom.

Personal stories present a means of revealing the problems of everyday practice in an embodied and memorable way, rather than presenting lecture material taken from text-books. Even though text books can be useful

Table 14.2 A structure for solution-focused teaching and learning

Be explicit about power relationships in the classroom

The classroom is a microcosm of what gets enacted in broader health and social contexts.
Do not assume equality is easily gained. Encourage access to power strategies by discussing differences in roles, finding ways to moderate hierarchy and make lectures dialogical

Generate dialogue

Dialogue is a practical way of making connections, of sharing knowledge, of exposing difference, of raising questions, of not accepting the rightness of the expert
Make a conscious attempt to make space for silent people to speak
Value diversity within the group, explore the tendency for people to seek sameness

Historicise current practices

Engage students in critical examination of the evolution of a current practice
From where did it originate, how it has changed over the years.
What forces have been molding it

Show how students can be critical

Explain differences between personal attack and critique of ideas
Model questioning behaviour
Show how to deconstruct textual information

Engage in knowledge play

Playing with language helps to reveal the dominant discourses hidden within them
Play can reveal how some groups have been silenced

Examine sites of resistance

Explore both conventional and unconventional practices
Discuss clients or service users who refuse the advice of experts
Who choose another path (e.g. acupuncture, homeopathy, religion)

Discuss ways of using privilege and power differently in health

In support of others
In working to create a just world
By showing compassion
By valuing diversity

resources, they can also be daunting and impersonal. Taking words from a page can teach many important things but may do little to engender an appreciation of the subjective realities of clients in students. Personal stories bring both the practising nurse and the consumer to life and situate the subjective experience as readily accessible to the student in the educational arena. This can provide a complementary subjective and social approach to the objective viewpoint of both text and teacher. Also, one of the key ways marginalized groups maintain their position is their silence. Storytelling is a means of vocalizing issues and perceptions that then become open to interpretation and understanding of the subjective.

Another strategy is to consider writing about the novel classroom approaches you have used. It is also useful to take any opportunity you can to co-teach and then co-write with colleagues. When you are working with a colleague, as I have done several times, you have the benefit of having someone with whom you can bounce around ideas, and also gain critical appraisal of your classroom teaching. Not only can this extend your skills, but it can generate enthusiasm and faith in the craft of teaching. Since I've managed to publish novel strategies several times, both on my own and with friends, I would like to share a few tips for those of you thinking of writing for publication on your teaching strategies.

1. Document your activities faithfully before and immediately following the classroom activity. This way your memory of goals, activities and achievements will be clear.
2. Locate your activity in the literature and in the local context. Provide description of the course, the population, its needs and resources. Explain how your idea is needed and novel. What significance does it have for the education of students, and the future better practice of clinicians? You need to impress upon the reader the relevance, meaning and potential impact of the intervention.
3. Evaluate the education intervention. Rich and meaningful evaluation data ideally combines qualitative data such as verbatim comments from students or stakeholders, as well as quantitative data such as descriptive statistics, changes in attitude, or observed changes in behaviour. Such data does not need to be elaborate or overly sophisticated. Simple trends and evidence of change will be relevant and informative.
4. Finally, use model papers to provide structure and inspiration. The Journal of Nursing Education frequently has good examples. Or search the work of Christine Tanner, Nancy Diekelmann, Philip Darbyshire or Phil Barker. I also suggest some of our own papers and provide a list for you at the end of the chapter.

By regularly sharing craft-knowledge of nursing education, we have the potential to extend the discipline and advance practice. As Nancy Diekelmann (1993) suggests, when we share our work and ideas publicly, we are being political. We create the potential for system change.

Table 14.3 The ABC model for planning lessons (McAllister, 2005)

A. A tone of interactivity, optimism and energy
B. Beliefs and perceptions about the issue are explored
C. Content
D. Demonstrated skills
E. Everybody practices
F. Family or friends recruited for support and invited to celebrate achievement

Searching for solutions also requires more imagination and creativity than the conventional problem orientation, which tends to privilege logic and reason. Thus, classroom activities can include lateral thinking, imaginative exercises which help students rethink the familiar, and think about the strange in novel ways.

Table 14.3 outlines my ABC model for planning a lesson. To illustrate how this model can be used effectively, consider how Susan approached a lecture on stigma. Not all ice-breakers and strategies to engage and inspire students work effectively in every context but you may find the strategies Susan used could be modified to suit your personal style and the needs of your classroom cohorts.

> Susan felt it might be a good idea to begin by involving the students. This would set an expectation for interaction and convey to students her belief that they had knowledge that could be shared. She began: 'There are all sorts of labels attributed to people in our society, based upon what you look like, or how you behave. (Susan paused). But not all of these labels are bad. Let me ask you … If you are male, tall, handsome, wearing a suit and tie, people might think you are … what?' (Susan got one or two quiet answers, and responded effusively to each of them).
>
> One student said, 'A lawyer?'
>
> Another, 'A male model?'
>
> One wise guy suggested, 'Johnno!'
>
> And Susan responded, 'Ok, right! How about this one, if you are female, slim, wearing a midriff top with a belly button ring, people might think you are … ?'
>
> This time, the question aroused many answers, some from belly-button ring wearers themselves, warding off any attacks on their identity.
>
> She continued, 'So, when these labels lead to negative judgments that's stigma. Stigma is a shameful sign of difference. It affects identity, and its impact can be reduced.' (Susan wanted to explain the whole idea of stigma and how it can be moderated. She wanted to emphasize an optimistic tone i.e. (A).
>
> Susan then set about uncovering students' beliefs about stigma (B).
>
> She asked, 'What comes to mind for you, when you think of stigma?'
>
> By this stage, it wasn't hard to generate lively conversation because students were now ready to have their say. Susan had often found it didn't take much to open students once an interactive tone had been established at the outset.
>
> Susan eventually moved to the next stage of the session and gave what she thought would be some interesting background information about stigma – the existing

knowledge on the subject. She provided a definition. She outlined sources of stigma such as myths, taboos, labeling, having a disability-focus. She drew on Sander L Gilman's work on representations of illness (1988). She discussed, using different cultural groups, historical changes, the consequences for the stigmatized person and the forms that stigma can take. Finally she pointed out literature recommending social solutions for overcoming stigma. (C)

With one third of the time remaining, Susan wanted to stop delivering content and once again engage the group.

She asked, 'Would you like to have a go now yourselves at working with a 'client' to help them work across stigma and labeling?' (Susan was met with a resounding yes. She knew from experience that students were eager for a chance to get in and practice).

So Susan continued, 'Since stigma is such an identity-stripping experience, it is useful to counteract that by engaging clients in work that: builds up their identity; helps them to see their resting strengths and resources; puts into context the idea that stigma is actually somebody else's problem – the person who holds the fixed beliefs. Now group together in pairs and play the 'who am I game' (see Table 14.4). You might see that this is an activity you can later do with clients]. (D)

Susan allowed the class to engage in some raucous activity where everybody got the chance to practise an activity they might one day use with clients. Susan used the time to go around and join in with the laughter. Occasionally she would reiterate the point about it being identity-building not stripping. (E)

Susan continued, 'And now to finish up. If we are serious about doing something to moderate stigma, then we need to focus not just on the client, but on families and friends. I thought of this idea and I'd like you to critique it.'

Once a client has engaged in the identity building game with you, you could use some humour by awarding them with a 'note of progress' that they could keep or show to their family/friend. It could read 'Congratulations! You have now talked about and noticed things about yourself that are positive and strong'.

A student commented, 'I think that's great, but you'd have to be careful that the client didn't think you were being patronizing'.

Another suggested, 'You could also give them a little affirmation card to remember the game or to pass on to others. It could say something like "I am more than my label." '

One other said, 'Yes, or it could read "Warning. All labels can pass their use-by date." '

Ideas for working across stigma continued for a few more minutes until the lecture time was over. In the end, Susan thought the ABC model for lesson planning went very well. She got the students engaged and thinking. She gave some content information and still had plenty of time for skills practice and critique.

Table 14.4 Who am I?

The game comprises 6 questions that help to get to know a person better.

1. What's your nickname?
2. What's your favourite movie?
3. What's your favourite meal?
4. What's your favourite song?
5. If you could wake up tomorrow with a new skill what would it be?
6. Name and explain four guests you would like to have to dinner

Evaluating and Researching the Teaching of Solution-Focused Nursing

The overall aim of a solution-focused classroom is for students to have a growing familiarity with and belief in solution-focused nursing. That is, they have an enhanced:

- Ability to understand the philosophy, components and practices of SFN
- Capacity and competence in enacting SFN
- Communication with others so that SFN becomes sustainable and the word is spread to others

So when you have evidence that students are working with and for clients, then you can have confidence that learning outcomes have been achieved. Working with and for clients may involve helping him or her to:

- Understand their diagnosis/label
- Talk about the problem, issues and needs confidently with health professionals
- Understand causes, triggers, soothers, treatments and social factors relevant to the issue
- Develop skills to change
- Acquire resources, social supports and motivation to maintain that change

Selecting methods that will measure and understand what worked within these interactions can be quite a challenge. The fundamental question that most educators and stakeholders want to ask is, 'What works in what context, with which group and at what cost?' Since groups of people each have different needs, circumstances, personalities and resources, one simple research method is unlikely to fit in every context. However, it is possible to design a rigorous educational evaluation design that avoids response bias, achieves high response rates and uses measures that have validity.

Wilkes and Bligh (1999) suggest the following principles for planning evaluation:

- Explore both process and outcomes of learning
- Measure multiple outcomes, such as: students' reactions, learning, changes in behaviour, and benefits to clients and carers
- Use qualitative and quantitative methods: to measure factors and illuminate understanding about educational experiences

Designing research that will extend the discourse of Solution-Focused Nursing is also a challenge, but necessary to build an evidence base and to show that (and how) the practice contributes (or not) to health outcomes. Table 14.5 provides a structure to guide a process of strategic inquiry into Solution-Focused Nursing.

Table 14.5 Strategic inquiry into Solution-Focused Nursing

Targets and Tools	*Exploratory*	*Evaluative*	*Action Oriented*
Student/Nurse Teacher Client Nursing Society Survey Interview Observations Narratives Diaries Documents Discourses Texts	• What is the personal experience of SFN? • How do specificu groups experience SFN? • What approaches are solution focused? • What processes are enabling of an SFN culture?	• What is the relationship between SFN and outcomes? • What are the boosters and barriers to SFN learning/practice? • What is the effect of a new SFN intervention?	• What resources are needed to enable SFN to develop? • How can SFN contribute to an anti-oppressive health culture?

Researching Solution-Focused Nursing in Practice

Social science research is crucial to the advancement not just of nursing but all practice disciplines. Such research offers the right equipment for mining and revealing all of those colourful, complex, diverse, unique experiences that embody what it is that nurses do. Numbers on their own do not do that well. As has been said once or twice before in this book nursing touches people. But how can that touch be weighed and measured accurately to persuade funding agencies to properly support it?

In keeping with the spirit of the both/and thinking and social justice ethos that characterize SFN, the following is proposed as a fitting framework to guide research (Table 14.6). As you will see, the framework encourages a mixed method design that utilises both the strength of numbers and the power of stories.

Table 14.6 Critical Social Theory Research Framework

Epistemology	*Sampling*	*Data Collection*	*Methods*	*Analysis*
• Inclusive agenda: Emancipatory, participatory, change oriented • Social and political lens: when one group in society has problems, these reverberate on other groups	• Viewpoints are diverse, some have not been heard, and need to be understood in political and cultural context • Objectivity/ balanced view is enhanced by exploring many viewpoints and being involved in the communities	• Uses mixed methods with community involvement • Aim is to facilitate positive change for the least advantaged • Questions are asked about the social aspects that	• Interpretive Phenomenology • Narrative Inquiry/ Analysis • Case Study • Appreciative Inquiry • Action Research • Collaboratives Practice • Development • Ethnography	• Discursive view, exploring power and social relations • Produces theory relevant to practice • Bringing about change in a social system is complex

Epistemology	*Sampling*	*Data Collection*	*Methods*	*Analysis*
• Attend to process as well as outcomes • Conscious of power & social justice	serve as barriers, rather than locating the issue within the individual	• Does not make claims that all problems have been solved • May raise questions about areas for change		

Solution-Focused Nursing may be a noble idea with potential to guide nurses and nursing, but without action it remains just empty theorizing. The next step is for it to be rigorously and repeatedly clinically proven.

Final Word

The insights, stories, solutions and strategies suggested in this book on Solution-Focused Nursing may not resonate for each and every nurse, nor may they remain relevant forever. But on behalf of all of the writers and people who inspired the narratives within this book, I do hope that you have been inspired to at least try something new. As Mary DeChesnay says, what's important is to stay creative and if one solution fails, then learn to fail successfully, by moving on to another. Einstein had similar thoughts, so I'll leave you with these two quotes to ponder:

- We can't solve problems by using the same kind of thinking we used when we created them.
- The important thing is not to stop questioning. Curiosity has its own reason for existing.

Teacher notes to accompany this chapter can be found at www.palgrave.com/nursinghealth/mcallister

Suggestions for Further Reading

Barker, P. (2002). The tidal model: The healing potential of metaphor within the patient's narrative. *Journal of Psychosocial Nursing and Mental Health Services, 40*(7), 42–50.

Barker, P. (2002). *My cousin Vinnie.* Accessed on the web on 06/06/05 at www.clan-unity.co.uk/my_cousin_vinnie.htm

Darbyshire, P. (1995). Lessons from literature: Caring, interpretation and dialogue. *Journal of Nursing Education, 34*(5), 211–216.
Diekelmann, N., Swenson, M. and Sims, S. (2003). Reforming the lecture: Avoiding what's already known. *Journal of Nursing Education, 42*(3), 103–105.
McAllister, M., Matarasso, B., Dixon, B. and Shepperd, C. (2004).Conversation Starters: Reexamining and reconstructing first encounters within the therapeutic relationship. *Journal of Psychiatric and Mental Health Nursing, 11*, 575–582.
McAllister, M. and Rowe, J. (2003). Blackbirds Singing In The Dead Of Night?: Advancing Dialogue on the Craft of Teaching *Qualitative Health Research. Journal of Nursing Education, 42*(7), 296–303.
Tanner, C. (2002). Keep a story in your heart: A message to the class of 2002. *Journal of Nursing Education, 41*(6), 239–240.

References

Cummins, J. and Sayers, D. (1999). *Brave new schools – Challenging cultural illiteracy through global learning networks.* New York: St Martin's Press.
Diekelmann, N. and Schulte, H. (1993). Interpretive research and narratives of teaching. *Journal of Nursing Education, 32*(1), 5–6.
Einstein, A. Quotes accessed on the internet on 06/06/05 at http://en.thinkexist. com/ quotation/
Gilman, S. (1988). *Disease and representation: Images of illness from madness to AIDS.* London: Cornell University Press.
Indigo Girls. (2000). Hammer and a nail. In *Nomads, Indians and Saints.* Audio cd. Sony.
McAllister, M. (2005). Transformative teaching in nursing education: Leading by example. *Collegian, 12*(2), 11–16.
Parker, J., Gardner, G. and Wiltshire, J. (1992). Handover: The collective narrative of nursing practice. *The Australian Journal of Advanced Nursing, 9*(3), 31–37.
Wilkes, M. and Bligh, J. (1999). Evaluating educational interventions. *British Medical Journal*, 318, 1269–1272.

Index